To: Kelly

THE PATH TO PHENOMENAL HEALTH

AN INSPIRATIONAL JOURNEY TO VITALITY AND WELLNESS

SAM GRACI

Sam Graci

WILEY

John Wiley & Sons Canada, Ltd.

National Library of Canada Cataloguing in Publication Data

Graci, Sam, 1946 - The path to phenomenal health / Sam Graci.

Includes index.
ISBN-13 978-0-470-83671-2
ISBN-10 0-470-83671-7

1. Health behavior. 2. Health. I. Title.

RA776.9.G73 2005 613 C2005-903373-8

Production Credits:
Cover design: Natalia Burobina
Typesetter: Mike Chan
Cover photo: Karen Whylie/Coyote Photos

Printer: Printcrafters

John Wiley & Sons Canada Ltd
6045 Freemont Blvd.
Mississauga, Ontario
L5R 4J3

Printed in Canada

4 5 6 7 PC 14 13 12 11 10

CONTENTS

Contents

Contents

CONTENTS

Contents

CONTENTS

ACKNOWLEDGMENTS

Dedicated to

Karen Elizabeth Ann, who unfailingly supported, encouraged and skillfully guided every sentence to properly shape this book, and for the daily glasses of fresh, organic vegetable juices.

Stewart Brown, whose enthusiasm, encouragement, belief and true kindred spirit was responsible for this book's publication; Joe Graci, who provided daily, resourceful, timely and updated research articles that improved every chapter of this book; Purna Ma, for her crucial editorial input, clarity of thinking and uplifting presence; Lisa Chisholm, for her motivation, enthusiasm and skilled advice; and Tara Stubensey, for her expertise, support and inspiration.

Thanks to

Shanta Ma, Beth Potter, Naomi Kolesnikoff, Nicole Wall, Marie-Josée Labelle, Jean-Yves Dionne, Louise L. Hay, Crystal Andrus and Dianne Fidler, whose encouragement turned these dreams into reality and to William Faloon, a research peer and friend.

A very special thanks to

The exceptionally skilled and talented team from John Wiley & Sons Publishing: Robert Harris, Publisher, who inspired my writing from the very beginning; Joan Whitman, Executive Editor, for her endless patience and superb literary guidance; Elizabeth McCurdy, Project Manager, for her invaluable input and diligent attention; Valerie Ahwee, Developmental Editor, for her simply invaluable knowledge and skill at sharing it; Michelle Bullard, Copy Editor, for her expertise, enthusiasm and suggestions that helped to shape this book; Mike Chan, Typesetter; Meghan Brousseau, the talented Publicist; Karen Whylie, Cover Photographer; and so many others for their wonderful support!

Part I

RENEW

1

FEELING GOOD IS GOOD FOR YOU

BEGIN A JOURNEY OF SELF-DISCOVERY

Staying healthy and energized each day is a *"present time"* challenge.

The promise of renewed health, abundant energy and a satisfied life can pave the road to happiness for every human being. I want to encourage much, much more of it in your lifetime.

As human beings, our energy, intelligence and optimism are in dynamic balance with one another and our environment, and we can change, transform and renew ourselves at any time. Every decision we make may result in either regret or a miracle. I encourage you to choose the miracle of health, happiness and fulfillment to enhance the quality of your life.

Let go of all the restrictions in your life that prevent you from feeling happy and healthy. It is easy to become trapped in negative patterns of eating, sleeping, thinking and living. Harvard Medical School calls it the "staleness syndrome." The 100 trillion cells in your body and the daily choices you make are actually engaged in a continuous feedback loop—they cross-talk. That is, cells send and receive messages from the environment, telling the body what to do.

If you are willing to try new approaches and end negative restrictive behavioral patterns, you can renew and revitalize your physical, mental, emotional and spiritual well-being and feel good about yourself.

You can gain a completely renewed and different understanding of your mind-body system and achieve greater meaning, happiness, creativity, enthusiasm and purpose in life. Wonderful new opportunities will arise within the essence of your being. I encourage you to undertake the practical approaches in this book to replace dangerous life-destructive choices with rejuvenating life-supportive choices and thereby renew your lifestyle and state of mind.

My professional and personal experiences have taught me that optimum well-being, a sense of feeling fulfilled, happiness and health are a dynamic partnership between our mind and body. I am writing this book to inspire you to renew real dynamic balance in your life by opening the communication channels between your mind-body-mood-spiritual energy centers. They are the mind-body connection.

This book will give you the practical tools to experience immediate:

- renewed hope
- self-healing
- balanced living
- enhanced moods
- dynamic energy

THE MIND-BODY CONNECTION IS POWERFUL

An optimistic and happy outlook is the best way to stay healthy. Feeling good isn't just a vague feeling, it's a physical state of the brain, one that you can induce deliberately. It would appear logical that the link or connection between your mind and body would bolster well-being in general. People with an optimistic, happy brain develop about 50 percent more antibodies than average in response to flu vaccines. That is a significant difference.

Doctors have known for years that clinical depression—the extreme opposite of happiness—can worsen heart disease, diabetes, digestion, sleeplessness and skin tone, and lead to a host of illnesses. The mind-body connection between heart disease and clinical depression is surprisingly similar. Beneath the emotional surface of mood and depression can be a raging undercurrent of hormonal imbalances, impaired immunity, and inflammation. Depressed people, in fact, suffer a 400 percent greater risk of heart attack.

Other recent studies have discovered that hopefulness, optimism and contentment appear to reduce the risk or limit the severity of cardiovascular disease, pulmonary disease, diabetes, hypertension, colds and flus.

People who feel good or optimistic see life, physical health and mental wellness as a gift, so they are more willing to maintain their health and take better care of themselves than sad people do. Gratitude has been proven to boost your immune system and your good mood staying power, and help you stay healthy and actually live longer.

Dr. Candace Pert, director of the Brain Biochemistry Division at the National Institute of Mental Health, has pointed out that it is quite arbitrary to say that a neurotransmitter like "good mood" serotonin or "energizing" dopamine belongs to either the body or the brain. These neurotransmitters are as much sheer intelligence as they are physical matter. Dr. Pert refers to this "network of information" as the mind-body connection. The mind-body connection is gaining long overdue credence and a degree of respectability that will ultimately make everyone much healthier and happier.

THE MIND-BODY CONNECTION IS A POWERFUL INFINITY LOOP

INFINITY LOOP

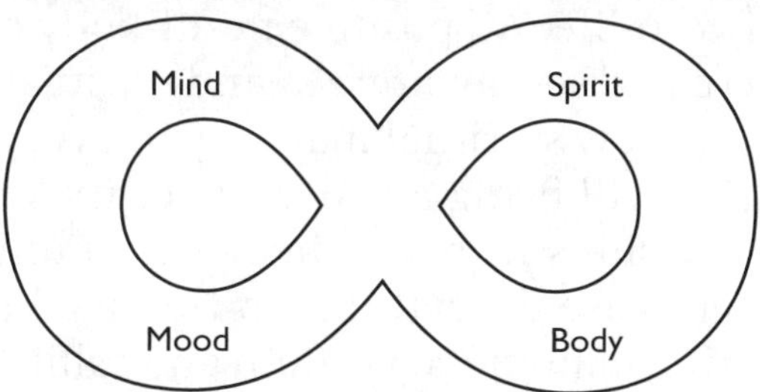

Your powerful mind-body-mood-spirit energy centers are the critical regulators of the flow of your vital life force. Positive signals anywhere in the dynamic mind-body-mood-spirit infinity loop affect the whole and remove unnecessary restrictions. Your experiences resonate in all four centers. You cannot be happy or sad, awake or asleep, sick or well, energetic or lethargic without sending a message everywhere within and along the infinity loop's circuit.

If there is anything you want to change, you can start with a positive signal anywhere on the loop and proceed from there. Because we are rooted in the material world, however, it may be easiest to begin by making small changes, such as how we eat or breathe. A simple change in diet can send signals so that you feel more energetic and have better concentration, and can even boost your good mood and joyfulness. Meditation, prayer and laughter improve your disposition, happiness, enthusiasm, immune system and work productivity. This is why I encourage you to start positive change in any aspect where you feel comfortable changing. All positive interventions send positive signals to and along your entire infinity loop so that all your cells receive a renewed message of positive transformation.

ACKNOWLEDGE YOUR SPIRITUAL CONNECTION

As you become aware of your infinity loop, all your circuits will turn "on." As you transform the familiar mind-body-mood circuit, your spiritual circuit will open. The need for a genuine spiritual interpretation of and involvement in life is universal. You will become more aware of the inner guidance at work in your life. You will begin to care for your spirit as consciously as you now care for your physical body—everything will then have spiritual value.

Your spiritual thoughts and activities are inseparable from other aspects of your life. All positive mind-body changes enable you to attain increased self-awareness and spiritual maturity. You will integrate your new spiritual maturity in everyday decisions. Spiritual maturity will bring a sense of clarity so that you will begin to make decisions from the heart and not just the mind. You will no longer base everything on the need to survive, but on the need to bring happiness, wisdom and fulfillment into your life each day.

When we begin to live with our mind-body connections in balance, we do not blame other people for our challenges. Instead, we realize that something is trying to wake up inside of us. Life's challenges are only a way of prompting us to become more self-aware—please wake up.

The awakening requires the energy self-management skills of "cell-friendly" foods, stress reduction, deep breathing, emotional balance, meditation and self-examination so that potent energies within us can emerge. Each of us has a special gift to offer. When we allow the mind-body-mood-spiritual energy centers to open equally, each of us is inevitably led to our own holistic path.

WANTING TO FEEL GOOD IS IMPORTANT—BUT THERE IS NO SUBSTITUTE FOR ACTION

Every positive choice you make is a good one and sparks an increased, powerful energy current in your life. To be effective, a change or new step does not have to be big. Making healthier food choices, meditating or adding an exercise regime is a good beginning. You could start walking every day; take a hatha yoga, Pilates or Tai Chi class; or learn to be optimistic. Along the way, continue to read up on all the information that expands your knowledge about what it takes to increase your robust vitality all day long, all life long.

Read books about alternative health options, and experiment with some of the practical suggestions immediately. If you feel you need group support, go to a neighbourhood health food store or holistic health resource center and check out the support groups in their listings or on the bulletin board. If you feel that a friend or nutritional therapist would be helpful, seek one out. You can make all these changes while you are in the process of seeking additional advice.

Bear in mind that any healing, transformation or good change is above all a learning experience. Be a good student in pursuit of human excellence. Above and beyond all, remind yourself as often as is necessary, each and every day, that you can't afford to fall prey to the, "Oh! I'll start tomorrow" way of thinking. Learning to renew your robust vitality, enthusiasm, optimism, self-esteem and spiritual grandeur is always a "present time" challenge and there is only "now" in any healing process. To the unconscious mind, time is irrelevant. Tomorrow, as they say, never really comes!

Begin to live today knowing that *today's* choices will determine *tomorrow's* future you.

Now you can fulfill your life's purpose and enjoy a happy, satisfied life.

FINDING YOUR HIDDEN SELF—THE GIFT OF CHANGE

Unquestionably, you do have true freedom—the freedom to take charge of yourself, to remove your anxiety and distress. You may have had challenges in the past such as low self-esteem, embarrassment, pain, anxiety, fear or failures that now challenge and influence your ability to see yourself as a person of robust vitality, happy, optimistic and bursting with inspiration. Your quality of life will improve when you clearly identify your current emotions and beliefs, which are either encouraging or limiting. Recognize the need to change any restrictive emotions or beliefs that are feeding self-destructive behavioral patterns. You need to identify what beliefs, perceptions and emotions will empower you to change your life.

When you recognize what positive emotions and dreams encourage, motivate and invigorate you, then you begin to experience real freedom—the freedom to transform yourself. It takes determined commitment and practice to reinforce your new enlightened beliefs and positive emotions. Continually focus on and remind yourself of your newfound emotions and beliefs to discover your enormous hidden personal power. Change your negative emotions of anxiety, stress and fear to calm, joy and fulfillment. Tell yourself that, "No matter what challenges I face on my path to optimum wellness, I will succeed in transforming myself from ordinary to remarkable." "I do enjoy taking good care of myself." "I now choose to live a life that reflects my awakened commitment to healthy food, conscientious living, emotional wellness and spiritual fulfillment."

"Believe that your life is worth living, and your beliefs will help create that fact."

William Blake

THE FOUR ENERGY CENTER REGULATORS OF PHENOMENAL WELL-BEING AND ROBUST VITALITY

1. a positive lifestyle ....for mind-body control
2. a healthy, cell-friendly diet ...for robust vitality
3. emotional wellness ....for great moods
4. spiritual fitness ....for inspiration

These four energy centers or circuits are your supercritical power centers for renewed healing, dynamic energy, joy, happiness and a satisfied, meaningful life. I call them the mind-body-mood-spirit centers. These centers, located in each of your one hundred trillion cells, are critical regulators for the flow of your vital life-force energy—your personal power. You are meant to discover both your extraordinary personal power and your shared purpose for being part of the human experience.

You must willingly and consciously bring awareness and attention, every day, to the challenges you face. Pay attention to how you respond to these challenges, and how you engage each center to experience optimum personal power.

You must see that truth is being delivered to you through these challenges or opportunities to grow and transform. You must also learn how to avoid being sapped or zapped by your own attachments, by other people's negative energy and by anything else that may be draining your intellectual, physical, emotional or spiritual power. Your body may be telling you loudly and clearly that you must re-evaluate your life. Ultimately, we must all leave behind our outmoded, limiting beliefs and behaviors, and creatively see ourselves in new, healthy ways.

Mind-body techniques may not cure a dilemma, but they make living with it a whole lot easier.

PSYCHOLOGY AND RESEARCH—EVEN THEY MUST GROW AND CHANGE

For most of its history, psychology has concerned itself with what makes the human mind unhappy and dissatisfied: anxiety, chronic stress, paranoia, depression, obsessions. The goal was to bring patients from a negative, ailing state to a neutral norm, or, as University of Pennsylvania psychologist Dr. Martin Seligman puts it, "from a minus five to zero."

Today we are not satisfied with just nullifying disabling conditions and getting to zero. We must explore how we can get from zero to plus five.

Hungarian-born psychologist Mihaly Csikszentmihalyi has explored a happy state of mind that he calls "flow," the feeling of complete engagement in a creative or playful activity familiar to poets, artists, musicians, athletes, deep thinkers, naturalist and meditation enthusiasts—almost anyone who loses himself/herself in a favorite pursuit. The concept of flow resulted in an explosion of worldwide research on happiness, optimism, positive moods and healthy character traits.

AUTHENTIC HAPPINESS—FEELING GOOD

In his book *Authentic Happiness,* Seligman writes, "I think we are our memories more than we are the sum total of our experiences." He finds three components to happiness: pleasure, engagement (the depth of involvement with one's family, friends, work, romance, hobbies and faith) and meaning (using personal strengths to grow and become more aware and mindful).

Of these three pathways to a happy, fulfilled, satisfied life, pleasure is the least consequential, he insists. This is important because so many of us build our lives around pursuing pleasure. Surprisingly, it turns out that engagement (being involved with the challenges and changes in your life) and meaning (finding your personal power and spiritual root) are much more important.

We can raise or lower our happiness and satisfaction levels significantly. What makes us happy and satisfied in life—wealth, education, youth, sunny days? Take wealth, for instance. University of Illinois psychologist Dr. Edward Diener, founding father of happiness research, has shown that once your basic needs are met, additional income does little to raise your sense of satisfaction with life. A good education? Neither education nor a high IQ pave the road to happiness. Youth? No again! In fact, older people are more consistently satisfied with their lives than the young.

MEASURE YOUR HAPPINESS

Diener devised the Satisfaction with Life Scale.

SATISFACTION WITH LIFE SCALE

Read the following five statements. Then use a 1 to 7 scale with 1 being not at all true, 4 being moderately true and 7 being absolutely true to rate your level of agreement.

1. In most ways my life is close to my ideal.
   ① ② ③ ④ ⑤ ⑥ ⑦
2. The conditions of my life are excellent.
   ① ② ③ ④ ⑤ ⑥ ⑦
3. I am satisfied with my life.
   ① ② ③ ④ ⑤ ⑥ ⑦
4. So far I have received the important things I want in life.
   ① ② ③ ④ ⑤ ⑥ ⑦
5. If I could live my life over, I would change almost nothing.
   ① ② ③ ④ ⑤ ⑥ ⑦

TOTAL SCORE________________

Scoring:

- 31 to 35: you are extremely satisfied with your life
- 26 to 30: very satisfied
- 21 to 25: slightly satisfied
- 20: neutral
- 15 to 19: slightly dissatisfied
- 10 to 14: dissatisfied
- 5 to 9: extremely dissatisfied

TWELVE "FEELING GOOD IS GOOD FOR YOU" BOOSTERS

Want to immediately boost your level of feeling good? Your energy levels will soar when you incorporate into your life these practical suggestions based on recent research findings.

1 **Let life's joys linger.**
Pay close attention to all your daily wonders and pleasures. Some psychologists recommend taking "mental photographs" of happy moments to review in less happy times. Sit quietly, rock in a rocking chair, lie on the grass and look up at the clouds, play with your children, adopt a pet, visit your parents, grandparents or friend, volunteer for a cause you believe in. Maintaining joy and wonder in life is an antidote to feelings of fear and inadequacy.

2 **Learn to forgive.**
Let go of any resentment or anger, perhaps by writing a letter of forgiveness, to a person who has wronged or hurt you. Forgiving allows you to move on, while dwelling on revenge poisons your mood, attitude and disposition, wrinkles your face and destroys both your physical energy and mental well-being. Forgiveness is a self-management technique to ensure you have a peaceful heart.

3 **Daily meditation and prayer.**
These are the best ways to raise optimism, hope and positive attitudes to life. Daily meditation and prayer are powerful ways to boost your moods by raising your "youth hormone" dehydroepiandrosterone (DHEA), reducing the acidic and corrosive stress hormone cortisol and boosting your "feel good" neurotransmitters dopamine and serotonin in your brain.

Religious or spiritual people are less depressed and less anxious. They are better able to cope with such crises as illness, pain, divorce, bereavement and loss of a job. Doing good works through acts of charity, compassion and prayer provides a sense of authentic spiritual connectedness and grounding. Love, faithfulness and hope are all linked to real happiness, gladden the heart and keep us open to the miracle of life. Meditation and prayer restore a healthy relaxed rhythm to the nervous system and to your heart. When you relax, your nervous system tunes down brain waves from the frazzled beta waves, to the alert but peaceful alpha waves.

4 **Take time for family, friends and community.** The single biggest factor in your satisfaction with life appears to be strong, loving, personal relationships. Be a good and faithful family member, friend and world citizen.

5 **Count your blessings.** Keep a "gratitude journal" in which you write down three to five things for which you are currently grateful—from the mundane to the magnificent. Do this every evening for immediate long-term results and to build positive character traits like thankfulness and empathy.

6 **Practice acts of kindness.** You can practice both systematic (such as helping your aging neighbor) and random (such as letting the busy mom go ahead of you in the check-out line) acts of kindness. It gives you a true sense of connection with others; it makes you feel good, and generous and capable; it brings you smiles and causes both a chain reaction of reciprocated kindness and honor in relationships. Share!

7 **Take care of your physical well-being.** Eat cell-friendly foods that energize you. Get lots of fiber, exercise five days a week, use modern food-based supplements, get plenty of sleep, drink lots of water and green tea, walk daily and stretch like a cat. Eat organic food when possible. Be grateful for your healthy food and say a grace or thanksgiving before eating. Sit down to eat and savor your food.

There are ways to tweak your immune system with cell-friendly foods: dry red wine contains resveratrol, which has cardiovascular benefits; garlic contains nutrients that kill nasty pathogens; broccoli and cauliflower contain indole-3-carbinol and sulforaphane, which have cancer-suppressing compounds; and curcumin, the yellow pigment in turmeric, an ingredient in curry, reduces heart disease, cancer and Alzheimer's. India has the lowest incidence of Alzheimer's in the world.

8 **Cope with stress and life's challenges.**
Optimism and faith have been clinically proven to help people cope, overcome hardships and keep hope alive, especially during times of pain. Slow deep breathing, acupuncture, exercise, Tai Chi, hatha yoga, relaxation therapy, massage, saunas and quiet time reduce stress. Judgment and criticism are self-defeating. Learn to identify your triggers and develop techniques for self-management. Relaxation techniques on CD or DVD help reduce stress, as does listening to relaxing music, trying homeopathy or going for a walk without a destination. There is nothing like stress to fast-forward the aging process. Perhaps it is time to unclutter your bedroom, storage area, spare room, garage, kitchen or office. Rather than sell your "excess," pass it on to a family or person in true need.

9 **Seek out a Wise Elder.**
Express your appreciation to someone that you owe a debt of gratitude to: a parent, a child, a grandparent, a friend, a companion, a counselor, a teacher, your church leader, your prayer or meditation group, or someone who helped to guide you through one of life's crossroads. The "three blessings" exercise is a technique to take the time and briefly write down a trio of things that went well that day and why. Focus on such human strengths and virtues as gratitude, love, kindness, humor, curiosity, and eagerness to change, grow and transform.

10 **Be persistent. Be committed. Be tranquil.**
Life is characterized by impermanence and constant change. If you can pay close attention to daily changes in your life and self-manage them, you will have lifelong emotional joyfulness, peace, equanimity and spiritual maturity. Listen quietly to your own inner voice for guidance and direction. The spin-off is that you will experience better concentration.

11 **Invest time to breathe, smile and laugh.** Breathing deeply and slowly, smiling and genuinely laughing can enhance your mood instantly. Practice them daily. They can help you to cope with changes and make you both happy and content all day long. Laughter reduces the red-alert stress hormones cortisol and adrenaline by 70 percent and immediately increases your "feel good" neurotransmitters serotonin and dopamine, and the neuropeptide beta-endorphins by 40 percent, which keep us happy, receptive and approachable.

12 **Recycle and care for the environment.** Surprisingly, mindful, conscientious awareness of the environment can make you feel responsible, capable and connected to Mother Nature, and enhance social esteem. Use natural body care products and biodegradable home cleaners. Wash your clothes with biodegradable soaps. Recycle paper, glass, tin cans, tetra packs and cardboard. Feel part of the global ecology. Recycle paint and used oils. Take leftover prescription medication back to your pharmacy.

ACTIVE PEOPLE FEEL GOOD

Regular exercise can strengthen your brainpower as well as your muscles, and studies show it is a powerful mood booster. It is clear that your moods can affect your physical health, but can physical activity affect your mental health? Hippocrates thought so. He encouraged melancholy Greeks to get out and walk, and modern science proves that getting up off the couch may help some people as much as Prozac or psychotherapy.

> The benefits of exercise accrue quickly, but require constant reinforcement—so exercise five days a week.

Carl Cotman, director of The Institute for Brain Aging and Dementia at the University of California, Irvine, points out that exercise can improve anyone's mood and mental performance and make us happier and sharper at any age. It is free, it is fun and it doesn't take a whole lot of time.

Surveys of children or adults conclude that active people are much happier than couch potatoes, and less prone to illness, fatigue and depression. McMaster University researchers confirm that in a group of depressed patients placed on an exercise regimen, 60 percent got better in four months—the same proportion that recovered on antidepressants. And though 30 percent of the medicated became depressed again within ten months, only 9 percent of the exercisers relapsed.

THE WONDERS OF EXERCISE—BOOST YOUR MOODS

Besides improving circulation, building lean muscle mass and burning fat, exercise brings on an array of chemical changes in the brain. It boosts the activity of mood-enhancing, "feel good" neurotransmitters such as dopamine, acetylcholine and serotonin. Surprisingly, exercise increases the production of brain-derived neurotrophic factor (BDNF), a chemical that helps neurons multiply and form new connections. A bigger circuit board means better brainpower for life. Studies show that even ten minutes of vigorous exercise can trigger the release, and raise beta-endorphin levels for a full hour so you feel good, positive, happy and enthusiastic. One hour of exercise, both cardio and strength-building, raises beta-endorphins for 8 to 10 hours and enhances a healthy libido.

So pick an activity you enjoy and stick with it. You really have nothing to lose except a few extra pounds, fogginess, depression, regret and sorrows. Exercise, even brisk walking, for sixty minutes a day, will make you feel good, and feeling good is good for you.

In February 2005, the journal *Neurology* reported that those who engaged in regular physical activity in early adult life lowered their risk for Parkinson's disease by 60 percent compared with those who did not. Dr. William Evans and Dr. Irwin Rosenberg, from Tufts University, have documented that regular exercise lowers the risk of osteoporosis and heart disease by 60 percent. Furthermore, recent research proves exercise lowers the risk of Alzheimer's disease by 50 percent because the brain actively breaks down beta amyloid tissue (sticky, gooey proteins) rather than accumulate it in brain tissue. *The Journal of the American Medical Association* published research in May of 2005 that regular exercise cut the risk of breast cancer by 50 percent and if you do not smoke or drink alcohol, the risk plummets by a remarkable 70 percent.

RECOMMIT EVERY DAY TO FEELING GOOD

I'll quote Oprah Winfrey here. She was asked how she runs 5 miles a day, and she said, "I recommit to it every day of my life." I know happiness and satisfaction are like that. Every day you have to renew your commitment to be willing to grow, change and transform by practicing the twelve feel good boosters. These strategies will become habitual within twenty-one days if followed wholeheartedly.

A healthy adult's brain contains approximately 100 billion neurons. The loss of neurons is drastic in dementia or Alzheimer's, but no big deal in healthy individuals. Dendrites, the connection extensions between neurons—if fed a steady diet of cell-friendly food and new learning experiences—can flourish in the brain's critical information-processing sector throughout our forties, fifties, sixties, seventies, eighties, nineties and beyond.

Five essentials to keeping well in your forties to nineties and beyond: diet, exercise, challenge, novelty and love. Nutrition's importance is obvious. Exercise and stress reduction are also vital to the cardiovascular and respiratory systems that keep your brainpower going all life long. Being kind, happy, optimistic and challenged are equally critical to well-being.

BECOME A MASTER OF LIFE—FEEL FULFILLED AND EMPOWERED

Dr. Gene Cohen, author of *The Creative Age*, has been conducting a study of three hundred senior citizens. Half are participating in a community-based arts program, while the others serve as a control group. The members of the creative arts group, who are being challenged mentally, make far fewer visits to the doctor, use less medication and are less depressed, and are more optimistic and happy. Why? "You have a personal sense of mastery," says Cohen. Many other studies have shown similar results—feeling good is good for you.

Imagine recruiting all 100 billion of your brain cells right now—deciding to transform your life once and for all from ordinary to remarkable to reshape and re-create your life. See change as a must—not as a should. This decision is the power of change. Use affirmations; tell yourself what you desire to hear from others.

"The mindset that got us into all of this trouble. . . is not the mindset we need to get us out."

Albert Einstein

The robust vitality, enormous energy, stable emotions, contagious optimism and the constant, spontaneous healing you desire and "the quality of life you really yearn for is within you," states Christiane Northrup, MD, author of *The Wisdom of Menopause*. It may seem far away, elusive or a distant, unachievable dream. The truth is you have the power to manifest your highest dreams, to achieve optimum wellness—and you have had that power within yourself all along. This book will show you how to take correct action to access your forgotten inner strength, learn how to take risks and master change.

Put simply, what you truly think and believe is what you become. This realization may be the greatest knowledge in your life and the most powerful guaranteed method to achieve optimum wellness, emotional stability, happiness, optimism and spiritual inspiration to help you attain your own greatness. Remember to maintain your sense of humor and perspective. As George Bernard Shaw put it, "Life does not cease to be funny when someone dies, any more than it ceases to be serious when someone laughs."

USE YOUR LIFE'S CHALLENGES TO LEARN AND GROW

"When you're in solitary confinement you're six feet under without light, sound, or running water, there is no place to go but inside. And when you go inside, you discover that everything that exists in the Universe is also within you. Within you is great power."

Rubin Carter, *The Hurricane*

THIS IS SERIOUS FUN

- As a nutritional and lifestyle researcher, I have determined that there is only one classification for human beings.
- There are only senior citizens or those in training to be.
- How seriously are you taking your training? Do you want to become a rapidly aging senior or a Wise Elder?
- Be determined to become a Wise Elder and lift high the love, dignity, joy and quality of life of every person you meet. Be proactive in the evolution of our species.
- Let them say of you, "Job well done."

LESSONS FROM WISE ELDERS

Historically, there have been many people who grew and transformed in their senior years. Leonardo da Vinci was painting in his late sixties; Michelangelo was sculpting in his eighties; Leo Tolstoy wrote "Where Love Is, God Is" in his late seventies; Winston Churchill was politically active in his nineties. Five Wise Elders!

Sister Esther Boor, a Catholic nun of Dr. David Snowdon's nun study on aging and Alzheimer's, took up ceramics after she retired at ninety-seven and sustained creative energy to make those extra years more fulfilling before her passing at age one hundred and seven in 2002. Ravi Shankar gave a brilliant concert on April 7, 2005 celebrating his 85th birthday.

My adopted grandmother, Shanta Ma, at ninety has a sharp wit, keen intellect, a wonderful curiosity for life and contagious good humor, with the most genuine heart-warming laughter. She meditates and prays daily for all humanity. Bea Nevill, my ninety-year-old good friend, is a pure delight. At eighty-seven she was arrested for blocking a logging truck. The judge said, "I can't put you in jail, you're my grandmother." At seventy-seven years young, my brother Joe Graci is a Wise Elder. One evening after a public lecture in Edmonton, Alberta, I returned to my hotel room and found a message on the telephone answering machine from Joe: "Sam, I just bought a new bench press yesterday and today I went cross-country skiing for the first time."

My father, Papa Joe, began the path to phenomenal health at the age of eighty-five with two major strikes against him. He had serious descending colon cancer and had to have twenty-two inches of his colon removed. The cancer had also spread to his liver. Besides that, Papa Joe had severe arthritis in his knees. His hair was white and quickly receding. He full-heartedly changed, living and eating by these recommendations. After seven days Papa Joe was a believer and after twenty-one days a devoted participant, and went on to live the best decade of his life, ten vibrant and healthy years from eighty-five to ninety-four. At ninety-four, the cancer in his liver brought this vibrant chapter of his life to an end. Papa Joe taught us how a Wise Elder should exquisitely expire. I held him in my arms while he shouted "I am ready, I am ready—I want to go home now," elegantly passing beyond the shores of life. With a lovely smile of equanimity and utmost peace he continued on his new journey. Job well done, Papa Joe.

THE PATH TO PHENOMENAL HEALTH

The path to phenomenal health is not a diet—it is a lifelong energy control program that will boost your energy, joy, self-esteem, good moods and brainpower for a healthy and happy lifetime.

The loyalty effort rewards you with immediate frequent-flyer miles including brainpower, emotional and energy upgrades.

2

POSITIVE THINKING DOES MAKE YOU HAPPY

The first step to any transformation is to change our perception, our outlook, our thinking—to renew ourselves. Every instant of your existence is an elegant dance of life.

So much of what we suffer is actually created in our own minds. We set the scene by how we react to the things that make us feel down, that stress us, that make us feel melancholy and zap our energy. Suddenly, pessimism or self-pity can make us even more angry, negative, depressed and tired of being tired.

If we have the courage to look at events more deeply, we realize that so many of the "bad" events in life—like the loss of a job or the end of a long-term friendship or relationship—can actually turn out to be blessings in disguise. We look back and realize that the majority of supposedly bad events in our life resulted in new learning, new perceptions and new challenges for personal growth. We must realize that even the death of a parent, child or other loved one, or a life-threatening illness, can be an opportunity for personal growth, change and positive transformation.

It is positive thinking that can keep any of us happy, growing and transforming our lives from better to better to better.

DO NOT BECOME A VICTIM OF IDENTITY THEFT

Knowingly or unknowingly, you have often shifted the neuromessengers in your brain, which control moods in your mind-body energy circuit, from one extreme to the other. The precise control to change and transform your awareness and perceptions—to access your dynamic personality potential—is within your direct control, even if it appears to be off the radar screen of your conscious thoughts.

When you are exceptionally happy, you are not the same person, physiologically speaking, as you are when you are mired in deep confusion or depression. The fine workings of the mind-body connection are very complex, but you can successfully alter your perception and use this powerful potential to transform for the better. When you are happy, the brain wave patterns on a roll of EEG paper as it rolls off the electroencephalograph are very different from the patterns your brain produces when you are sad. You are composed of both of these personality possibilities and many others.

We are not just a stream of consciousness framed into the description of 1990s pop psychology. We are not just mere physical bodies made of carbon, hydrogen, nitrogen and oxygen that have learned to think, but are intelligent thoughts that shape and reshape a physical body and brain.

We are designed with brilliant intelligence, enormous potential and a super-normal level of consciousness as a customized, built-in feature seldom explained in our owner's manual. This has come as a tremendous surprise to cellular biologists. You do not need to fill up your brilliant brain and unfathomable cosmic mind with more library-like knowledge, but with inspired insights and mind-body awareness. And for this you require only intentionality.

Expectations determine outcomes. When you upgrade your expectations of yourself, you are able to release any uncomfortable resistance and judgments you may have and revitalize your joy, enthusiasm and passion for living that will permeate all other aspects of your life. By expanding expectations of yourself and perceptions in your life, you become more receptive to new insights and visions, which will enable you to have a more spontaneous and creative response to life. This new insight and flexibility allows you, with unlimited creative potential, to resolve any challenge or dilemma that you may be facing. You can co-create your reality every moment with a creative and enthusiastic response by letting go of any limiting restrictions.

As my earlier story about the miracle of Papa Joe completely changing and transforming to a healthier lifestyle at eighty-five demonstrates, the miracle of human potential is that it is never too late to change and renew our perceptions, enthusiasm and passion for a happy life.

To your unconscious mind, time is nonexistent and irrelevant.

FEELING GOOD IS GOOD FOR YOU

In Chapter 1, "Feeling Good Is Good for You," I emphasized that you can change and transform your program, free yourself forever and be both healthy and happy. It is simpler than you may think because there is only one principle to reprogramming.

Principle: *As you think, so you are—and so you will be.*
Start by loving yourself. Start by being good to yourself. Start by doing for yourself all the things you do so well for your children, your partner, your parents and your friends. Take a detoxifying sauna followed by a massage. Go for a walk by the water or a hike in a park. Stay up just to watch the stars twinkle and the moon beam. Take up a craft, hobby, exercise class or sport, or take a course in something you always wanted to do. Go to an art gallery, an interesting museum, a zoo, a planetarium. Surprise a friend with lunch. Take the time to leisurely stroll through a library or store you really like. Go to a studio or outlet where local craftspeople and artists display their beautiful creations—admire and enjoy.

Stop on the street for a few minutes and enjoy the music of a good musician and acknowledge their work. Purchase tickets for a play, a movie, a ballet, a symphony, Cirque du Soleil or sporting event and surprise a person whom you know will be thrilled. Visit your grandfather or grandmother and just tell them "thank you."

Decide to do something that is fun, even for a short time, every day. Just walk into an open church, synagogue, chapel, mosque, temple or meditation spot and sit quietly, enjoying a respite from the noise and high technology. Listen to your inner voice. Listen to the buzz from your 100 trillion cells dancing, quiet, content, in balance and talking to you peacefully.

Remind yourself that life is full of ups and downs, and it cannot always be kind. Everyone's life is full of challenges. This is a fundamental truth. This has been, is, and always will be the nature of everyone's life.

The one true freedom you possess, whether you realize it or not, is that you can choose how to perceive and respond to difficult situations.

While attending university I set up a program for young offenders in jail. I was amazed one day when nineteen-year-old Pierre said, "Sam, I am learning to be happy to see, and grateful to have, this ray of sunlight that comes through my window. Prisoners on the north side don't have that." My friend James recounted that at eighteen years of age he was unnecessarily and viciously attacked by a trained police dog and had his face severely lacerated. He said to me, "Sam, that was a turning point in my life. I could have hated them forever, but I decided to forgive them; it is better for my heart."

We must remember that we can change how we respond to those dreadful and stressful times—from the routine, mundane daily events like waiting in a very slow-moving line at the grocery store to life- or health-threatening possibilities that hang over us.

Negative expectations actually breed negative experiences.

A positive attitude yields great returns in daily living because it helps you maintain optimum good health. Researchers like Deepak Chopra, Dr. Wayne Dyer, Lorna Vanderhaeghe, BSc, Dr. Larry Dossey, Caroline Myss, PhD, Louise L. Hay and Marianne

Williamson prove emphatically that the higher your optimism, the healthier your immune system. Positive expectations and optimism will lead to a self-fulfilling prophecy, making it more likely that good things will happen to you. Developing a positive attitude and staying balanced and content rather than giving into self-pity is hard, conscious, moment to moment, and continual work.

RENEW A POSITIVE RHYTHM TO YOUR HEART

Researchers at the Institute of HeartMath® (IHM) research center in Santa Cruz, California, are exploring the physiological mechanisms by which your heart communicates with your brain. They are eager to understand how the communication networks between your "feeling" heart and your "thinking" brain influence your perceptions, attitude, emotions, mood and overall health.

"If you think in positive terms you get positive results—if you think in negative terms you get negative results."

William James, psychologist

IHM researchers hope to learn why positive emotional states such as love affect you in a positive physiological way. Conversely, they want to learn how stress, worry, low self-esteem, anxiety and other negative emotional states harm your immune system, energy, heart, brain and hormones so that you become disheartened.

IHM researchers suggest that instead of always using your head, try visualizing, perceiving, feeling, and thinking from the heart. Send positive, loving and supportive feelings to yourself and others—it works. Physician and author Dr. Larry Dossey has proven that positive thoughts and sincere prayers emotionally, physically, mentally and spiritually help ourselves and others. When people point to themselves, they generally point to the heart.

Your heart rhythms are the best reflection of your inner emotional states. Positive emotions create increased harmony and balance in both the heart rhythms and nervous system. Negative emotions lead to increased disorder and imbalance in heart rhythms and the sympathetic nervous system.

EMOTIONAL SELF-MANAGEMENT

The HeartMath researchers have shown that you can combine positive feelings, such as compassion, gratitude, love and appreciation, with your breathing to effectively reduce stress and anxiety. Learning to send feelings and affirmations of love and gratitude throughout your system while breathing deeply allows a calmer heart to add new dynamic, positive emotions to your self-management and to your healing medical integrations. According to the main researcher Dr. Rollin McCraty, generating self-sustaining positive emotions helps you maintain emotional balance and alert awareness for longer periods, even during challenging situations.

> "Our modern western emphasis on the brain instead of the heart may be faulty. Leading with the heart may be the right way to go after all."
>
> Hyla Cass, MD, *Natural Highs*

RENEW A POSITIVE RHYTHM TO YOUR NERVOUS SYSTEM

Panic attacks destroy your heart and nervous system rhythms. They can happen during the day or night when no apparent danger is present. The surge in the panic attack hormones adrenaline and cortisol are the results of your sympathetic nervous system's (auto control) fight-or-flight response. When you live under long-term acute stress, your adrenal glands become overreactive and hypervigilant. With no forewarning, you can experience a pounding heartbeat, anxiety, feelings of frustration, exhaustion, shallow breathing and feelings of impending doom.

To avoid panic attacks, which destroy your positive attitude, stop and breathe deeply and slowly. This slow breathing will restore a healthy rhythm to your nervous system by turning off your sympathetic and turning on your parasympathetic nervous system to buffer the surge of exaggerated cortisol and adrenaline, the red-alert hormones.

EXCELLENCE VERSUS PERFECTION

All too often the cause for failing to take good care of yourself with a healthy diet, or being committed to your personal transformation, meditation or regular exercise, is getting caught in perfectionism. True balanced living and optimum wellness are all about personal excellence, doing the best you can, trying to raise your standards each day, exercising your freedom and right to choose your best, and stepping up and showing up as your very best. If you find yourself being self-critical, finding fault with or not trusting yourself, please remember the voice within you. Ask for guidance and strength. Know for sure that creating a life of vitality and well-being is a process and not a destination.

Your new health experience and life are a continuous commitment to daily excellence and not perfectionism.

I received a beautiful letter from Jackie McKelvie of Saskatoon, Saskatchewan. I had recently met Jackie in Saskatoon when I gave a lecture at one of my very favorite nutritional stores—Dad's Nutrition. Fred, Jackie's husband at seventy-nine years young, is the oldest *Globe and Mail* newspaper delivery person in Canada. Fred fine-tuned his diet at seventy-eight and takes two scoops, one vanilla and one chocolate, of *proteins+* protein powder and makes a power shake to drink on his route.

Jackie is one of the finest people I have ever met. At seventy-nine she said, "Sam, I have a degree in nursing. I thought I knew so much, but I have learned so much from you, and we are making those changes."

Jackie and Fred pursue excellence.

HOW STRESSED ARE YOU? ARE YOU REACTING, OR ADAPTING?

You know when you are stressed, but you can obtain a more objective measurement of how much tension and anxiety you're experiencing and how much it is costing your mental, physical, emotional and spiritual well-being.

Two researchers at the University of Washington School of Medicine in Seattle, Thomas Holmes, MD, and Richard H. Rahe, MD, devised what has become the standard professional gauge of stress and the likelihood that it will cause you illness. Dr. Rahe and Mark A. Miller, PhD, updated the scale in 1997 and called it the Rahe Life Stress Scale. The Rahe Life Scale is from the *Journal of Psychosomatic Research* 43, 1997, and used with permission from Elsevier Science.

The World Health Organization has estimated that by the year 2020, depression due to stress will be so prevalent that only heart disease will affect a greater number of people. The Centers for Disease Control and Prevention in Atlanta stated in a March 22, 2005 *USA Today* story on stress that, "Up to 90 percent of doctor visits may be triggered by a stress-related illness."

The brilliant physician Hans Selye said, "Every stress leaves an indelible scar, and the organism pays for its survival after a stressful situation by becoming a little older."

The Rahe Life Stress Scale

Life event	Score
Death of a child	123
Death of a spouse	119
Death of a close family member	101
Divorce	96
Marital separation	79
Jail term	75
Fired from work	74
Serious illness	74
Death of a close friend	70
Pregnancy	67
Birth or adoption	66
Miscarriage or abortion	65
Major business readjustment	60
Major loss of income	60
Parents divorce	59
Relative moves in	59
Credit difficulties	56
Change in health or behavior of a family member	55
Retirement	52
Change to different line of work	51
Major decision about future	51
More arguments with spouse	50
Marriage	50
Parent remarries	50
Accident	48
Partner begins or ends work	46
Engagement	45
Sexual difficulties	44
Moderately severe illness	44

Birth of a grandchild	43	Change in work conditions	35
Loss/damage to personal property	43	Change in schools	35
Child leaves home	42	Trouble at work	32
Change in living conditions	42	Change in religious beliefs	29
Change in work responsibilities	41	Change in church activities	27
Change in residence	40	Change in personal habits	26
Personal relationship problems	39	Change in number of family get-togethers	25
Begin or end school	38	Change in political beliefs	24
Trouble with in-laws or relatives	38	Vacation	24
Major increase in income	38	Minor purchase	20
Major purchase	37	Less-serious illness	20
New close relationship	37	Minor law violations	20
Outstanding achievement	36	Taking courses	18

Interpreting Your Score

Check off the events you have experienced in the last year on the Rahe Life Stress Test. Add up the numbers attached to each one. This total shows your Life Change Units (LCUs). A score below 200 indicates that you have a low risk of a near-future illness. A score between 201 and 300 means your odds of getting sick are moderate. A score between 301 and 450 indicates a high-risk concern. Finally, if you score greater than 450, you are at a very high risk for imminent illness. This is why you must deliberately and consciously seek to counteract self-destructive stress with calmness, insight, deep breathing, meaningful pauses, prayer, meditation, laughter, humor and authentic joy.

SURVIVAL MESSAGES FROM INNER SPACE

In 1975, Dr. Alexander Leaf, a Harvard researcher, published *Youth in Old Age*, a book about the cultures he had studied around the world who lived long, energetic, healthy lives.

In 1978, Dr. Hans Selye, a McGill University researcher and endocrinologist, published his book *The Stress of Life*. Selye continued the work of early twentieth century scientist Walter Cannon about the ability of accumulated stress to cause excessive wear-and-tear, while depleting our robust energy on a daily basis. Selye coined the term "fight-or-flight response" to explain that when you encounter a threatening situation, a part of your involuntary nervous system becomes instantly and automatically activated to increase heart rate, blood pressure, rapid breathing, and alertness to stimulate the adrenal glands to secrete the red-alert alarm hormones adrenaline and cortisol.

The original purpose of the fight-or-flight response was to help humans survive in threatening situations, because the ability to react quickly to a threat helped our ancestors to survive in a dangerous environment.

Today, the fight-or-flight response is a negative-alert response that no longer serves you well. It easily activates when you are faced with a final exam, a critical work deadline, a long line of traffic, an interpersonal dispute or a confrontation with a co-worker with whom you have an unspoken rivalry. However, today neither fighting nor running away is a positive, healthy option.

There is a pressure to react, to survive, to do something immediately, but there is no way to release this intense energy buildup, which results in a very harmful state called acute stress. Stress is so powerful that some people, within minutes, have literally died from shocking news or fear, because their circulatory systems and heart collapse and shut down. The long-term consequences of a continually activated stress-alert response robs you of your robust energy, enthusiasm, optimum production and well-being.

Today you do not need the constant stress alert that enabled your ancestors to survive. To survive well today in a fast-paced, multi-tasking, stressful environment, you need a revolutionary calm-alert response or a relaxation response.

Rather than drain your body all day long of its vital energy in non-critical emergency responses, you need a new method to adapt—not one to react. Today, it is not "survival of the fittest" but "survival of the wisest." You need to decompress and learn to respond with a calm alertness; because you cannot continually react, you must adapt. Today, researchers are using high-tech instruments to elucidate the mind-body connections, proving that stress or desperation damage your system-wide health, especially your brain neurons, neurotransmitters and neuropeptides, your "biological cell phone."

FINDING SHANGRI-LA

There is no question that the cycle of life can be one of continuous positive transformation. At the right time, in the right season, you find yourself ready for a rebirth, a resurrection, a quantum leap in creativity and renewal. It is critical that we raise our awareness, so that we can collectively make choices born of new perceptions that allow ourselves, the human species and the global ecology to evolve. Jonas Salk, the biologist who developed the first polio vaccine, once said that for humans to survive as a species we must move beyond the Darwinian idea of "survival of the fittest" to a new paradigm, "survival of the wisest." Follow the "wise" road map that makes your life feel more meaningful. We have access to Shangri-la right now, right here—in our creative awareness and renewed perceptions.

KEEP A POSITIVE, YOUNG AND HEALTHY MIND

If your mind is old, your body will reflect it. A youthful mind is constantly open to new growth, eager for transformation or a quantum leap into creativity. It is better to be sixty years young than thirty years old.

Dr. Alan Logan states, "Neuroscientists are learning that the brain is an extraordinarily dynamic organ that is continuously reshaping itself." The cortex of the brain, which is less than one-fifth of an inch thick and covers 360 square inches, contains over 20 billion neurons (brain cells). Each of these neurons can have a communication network of over 10,000 connections with other cells throughout your brain. Dr. Logan adds, "The electrical signals, chemical neurotransmitters, neuropeptides and magnetic energy circuits in your brain are in perpetual flux, reflecting your food intake, moods, stress level and your sympathetic or parasympathetic nervous system dominance." Unquestionably, your brain literally thrives on novelty in order to survive and improve its biological structure and electrochemical wiring.

> "The ideals that have lighted my way, and time after time have given me new courage to face life cheerfully, have been Kindness, Beauty, and Truth."
>
> Albert Einstein

Surprisingly, all of your experiences happen in your mind, which is always growing and changing, shaping and reshaping itself.

It is never too early or too late to shape your brain's destiny and encourage growth of new brain cell connections, boosting moods while increasing memory and learning capacity. There is every reason to believe your brain can give you a lifetime of fulfillment and happiness. Unfortunately, the typical North American diet and lifestyle are not conducive to creating and supporting superior brains.

By thinking positive thoughts; staying emotionally stable; renewing your lifestyle; eating cell-friendly, brain-ready, healthy foods; and using therapeutic natural supplements, you can keep your mind and body fresh, revitalized and youthful. A brain that is youthful is full of love, hope, enthusiasm, creativity, positive perceptions, spontaneity and spiritual maturity. This is the kind of high-impact change we all welcome.

Your brain is a wonderful treasure to be sculpted and nurtured throughout life—just what is needed to become a multi-dimensional Wise Elder.

3

ONE GREAT DAY EQUALS ONE GREAT LIFE

Living an outstandingly rich life with robust vitality, in dynamic balance and full of optimum wellness, *is your birthright*. Right now, at this very moment, you actually have the key to unlock your full potential and experience your life's fulfillment. When faced with a long "to do list," you can feel too overwhelmed and disheartened to be healthy and happy. Instead of allowing someone else to determine your list of things to do, what if you could choose all the great things to do today to attain the life of your dreams? What was the main message I tried to convey to teens at high risk? Just this: A small subtle change in your perception and belief will give you a profound change in outcome. I know it is worth the risk—I absolutely do.

Why be heavy? Be light!

Why feel heavy? Feel light!

Why have a heavy heart? Have a light heart!

Why eat a heavy diet? Try a light diet!

ONE NOT-SO-GREAT DAY

AN UNBALANCED DAY

To experience one dynamic day, you must be successful in creating balance in your day.

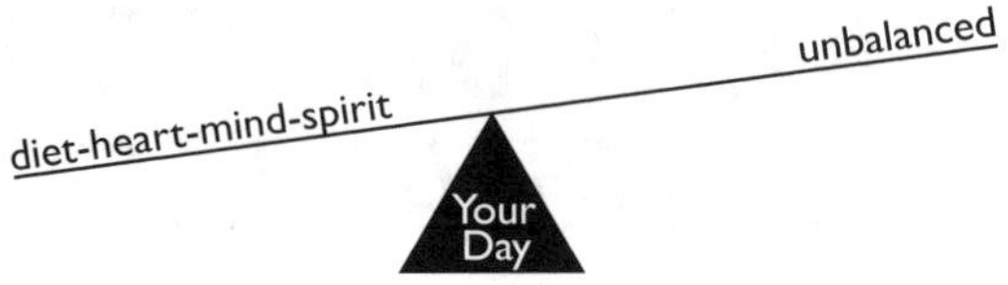

A heavy diet destroys your balance.
A heavy heart destroys your balance.
A heavy mind destroys your balance.
A heavy spirit destroys your balance.

A daily heavy diet, heart, mind and spirit = an unbalanced day.

Did you wake to your morning alarm, press the snooze alarm and get 5 extra minutes? Be perfectly honest. Ask yourself if that 5 extra minutes made a profound difference to your day. Will your day be a whole lot better for that 5 extra minutes or is a not-so-great day really due to denial, fear, lack of enthusiasm or just plain fatigue? Think of the alternative—you might not wake up ever again. Does it sound like scary stuff?

You may have to face yourself on this one. You may have to work this one out and discover who you are. Maybe it is time to stop being unbalanced, closed, caught in repetitive patterns and not really seeing every day as a new opportunity, a new challenge. It is time to change perceptions. Phillip C. McGraw, PhD, says that there is no reality—only perception.

ONE GREAT DAY
A BALANCED DAY

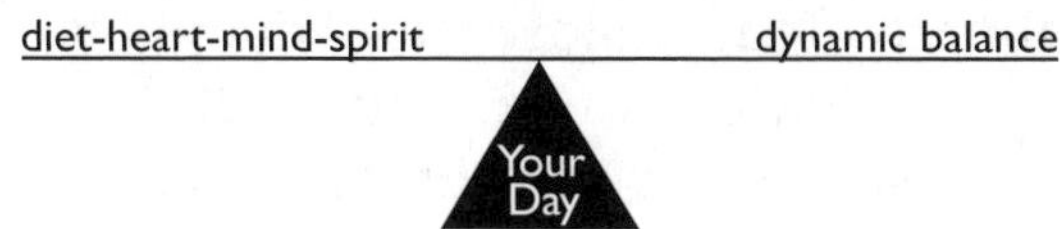

A light diet gives you dynamic balance.
A light heart gives you dynamic balance.
A light mind gives you dynamic balance.
A light spirit gives you dynamic balance.

A light diet, heart, mind and spirit = a dynamically balanced day.

You wake up feeling grateful for a night of deep, rejuvenating sleep. You feel refreshed, motivated and eager to experience the adventure of a whole new day. You breathe deeply, feeling the life-giving fresh air rushing into your lungs and you greet this new day as a new opportunity to grow, to learn, to experience, to change, to transform. You are ready to put your stamp of approval on the day.

Let's begin as soon as you wake up tomorrow morning. Do you wake up saying, "Good Morning, God" *or* do you wake up saying, "God, another morning!" Feel the phenomenal difference? Two different ways to start your day—one positive, one negative.

A very subtle change in perception and beliefs will give you a profound change in outcome—guaranteed.

SIX STEPS TO MAKE EACH DAY GREAT

First: As soon as you wake up, greet the day with utter gratitude. Deep sleep is a powerful prescription for rejuvenation. It also has many side effects—peace, equanimity, tranquility, simplicity in the moment, ease and a natural joy that you are alive! Let's face it—you won't be here forever, so have gratitude for this one day—today.

Second: Breathe very deeply and slowly, allowing your belly to balloon out and in. Breathe like this for six breaths. With each round of breathing in and out, think of one thing you are grateful for. Remember to breathe slowly and deeply, removing all the stale, acidic carbon dioxide waste, and refilling your lungs with fresh, alkaline, life-sustaining oxygen.

Third: Thank all the green vegetation on the earth and in the oceans for doing two critical jobs. In the Divine Blueprint, through the process of photosynthesis all green vegetation takes carbon dioxide, the toxic waste exhaled from your lungs, into its tissues as fuel and miraculously gives off pure oxygen—free of charge. The reason is irrelevant, just be utterly grateful and humbled that it does.

Fourth: Thank your parents, grandparents and great grandparents for the gift of life and tell them that on this one day, you will try hard to reverently and respectfully honor all their genes that have been passed on to you. Carry them with real dignity.

Fifth: Do what I do—"emergency open heart surgery." Upon standing, clasp your hands in front of your chest in prayer fashion, breathe in deeply and hold, then raise your clasped hands above your head, stretching as high as you can, lifting your shoulders, neck and head. Exhale slowly and evenly through both nostrils at the top of the stretch as you release your hands from above you and slowly allow your arms and hands to fall circularly to your sides. Repeat this breath six times, followed each time by an ear-to-ear smile.

Sixth: Stand quietly and alone for a minute. Initiate inner dialogue with yourself. Listen intently, calmly. Ask for guidance and direction. Ask for love and compassion. Tell yourself that you will make sincere contact with everyone you encounter that day: your mate, children, parents, brothers, sisters, housemates, workmates and all those you will meet in the course of your day. This sets the tone for both you and them to live the day well. When you do this, they will have a better chance to get to their destination safely and perform better. You will have conscientiously lifted them up and in doing so lifted yourself up.

CREATING BALANCE AND WELL-BEING

Everything we do comes back full circle to ourselves. That is the Law of Divine Recycling. Notice carefully how you feel throughout the day when you are truly acknowledged, appreciated and embraced. Your purpose, confidence and self-esteem are all empowered.

> "Think that every thought you think, every word you say plants a seed in the 'garden' of both yours and their life. Every word and every action plants a seed in our life to grow. To live the best you must plant the best."
>
> Nelson Mandela

Make sure that you truly connect, make contact and properly focus on each person, giving a nod, touch or hug before you move on. Express your passion for life to get what you need out of this new, unfolding day. Pay strict attention to your inner dialogue throughout the day. If your inner dialogue is not worthy of the precious genes you carry, or if the dialogue is not uplifting, change the tune at once. Don't ruin and poison this day from within. Several times throughout the day, stop and listen to see if your inner dialogue is full of critical negativity for others that could keep both you and them down—and let it go. Replace critical negativity with verbal, "critical loving" reinforcing phrases like "good for you," "congratulations," "have a very good day" and "wonderful."

PSYCHONEUROIMMUNOLOGY AND YOUR DAY

One statement I can make with total certainty is that there are direct pathways between your mind and your immune system. This fundamental concept—that you can proactively manage rather than reactively medicate your immune system—has led to a whole new field of Integrative Medicine that proves your immune system can be positively or negatively influenced by your mind. This science is called psychoneuroimmunology. The name refers to psychology (*psycho*, the brain), the nervous system (*neuro*) and your immune system (*immunology*). For example, high levels of stress and poor moods weaken your immune defences, making you more susceptible to colds and flus initially and resulting eventually in major problems such as heart disease and cancer.

A bad mood can quickly compromise your immune system. Positive thinking not only boosts your moods but maybe even saves your life by lowering corrosive, acidic cortisol and adrenaline and raising DHEA (your alkaline "youth hormone") and both dopamine (your "get energized" neurotransmitter) and serotonin (your mood-modulating neurotransmitter).

STRESS—A ONE-WAY TICKET TO A BAD DAY

You need a certain amount of daily stress to stay alert and motivated. But when your day is full of acute stress, you are creating a one-way ticket to a bad day.

> "Laughter is a tranquilizer with no side effects."
>
> Bob Marley, musician

Ron Nelson, forty-five, identified anxiety as a trigger for overeating and cut back on the pizza and Chinese buffets. "Before, I was on automatic pilot," he says, "and now I can take my time, eat healthy food and enjoy a smaller portion."

You have to learn self-management skills to deal with the continual stressors in daily life. Usually excessive stress unleashes mental images of traumatic memories. The stress response now becomes a red alert and the elevated anxiety lowers your emotional well-being. Ten hours later you can have difficulty falling asleep and for several days experience:

- depression, apprehension
- anxiety, fear, restlessness
- insecurity
- irritability, anger
- loss of libido
- impaired mood, foggy memory

ARE YOU ADDICTED TO THE ADRENALINE RUSH?

Nobel Prize winner Dr. Hans Selye, the father of stress research, proposed three stages to the stress response, which consists of alarm, adaptation and finally exhaustion. To stress is negative, to de-stress is positive.

If you begin to get hooked on the surge of addictive workaholic adrenaline and cortisol racing through your bloodstream, you need a new emotional response. When the stimulus of deadlines, constant duress and production stops, you can experience an adrenaline withdrawal and a pervasive feeling that you have to do something to boost stress and pump up the adrenaline rush. In these cycles, once you let go, you collapse in exhaustion, depression and a sense of worthless production. Your exhaustion becomes a case of emotional bankruptcy. Deep breathing and meditation will allow you to reduce and buffer the surge of exaggerated cortisol and adrenaline red-alert hormones and rebalance your adrenal glands.

Dr. Selye's three stages are:

1. **Alarm Stage:** In the red-alert phase, two tiny almond-shaped adrenal glands, one on top of each kidney, produce the stress-related hormones adrenaline, cortisol and DHEA. In a red alert, adrenaline kicks in immediately, then declines, but cortisol keeps going for hours. DHEA is released by the adrenals to reduce the stress and maintain your energy supply. High levels of DHEA increase new cell growth (neurons) in your brain, thus increasing memory, energy, intelligence, good mood and brain function. Low DHEA levels decrease libido, mood, energy and brain function. Elevated DHEA reduces the symptoms of menopause without ingesting synthetic estrogen and progestin drugs that have been shown to cause lethal side effects, according to the medical journal *Fertility and Sterility*.
2. **Adaptive Stage:** Corrosive cortisol and beneficial DHEA have a reciprocal relationship, so as cortisol levels go up, DHEA falls and vice versa. If cortisol levels dominate, you feel increased anxiety, fatigue and mood swings. If DHEA dominates, the stress and anxiety decline quickly and you boost your mood. Deep breathing and meditation increase DHEA and reduce both cortisol and excessive adrenaline rushes.

3. **Exhaustion Stage:** When you become stuck in the red-alert stress response, you wear out your ability to produce either cortisol or DHEA. Vital nutrients like vitamins and minerals become depleted, your get-energized hormone dopamine declines and your emotions slip into depression. In the 1990s, anti-anxiety medications called benzodiazepines ("benzos"), such as Ativan, Labrium, Xanax, Clonopin, Rhovane, Rivotril, Serax and Valium, became popular to treat anxiety, panic disorders, stress and insomnia. When they are burned out, people find it easier to take anti-anxiety medications than to deal with symptoms. Your adrenal glands are exhausted when you are burned out. If you choose to stop taking these medications, you must do so only under medical supervision, as a sudden withdrawal can cause severe reactions like seizures. Benzodiazepines have some value in assisting people through a brief period of acute stress but they have some side effects, including daytime fatigue, lethargy, nightmares and fragmented sleep. Benzos are designed to increase the synthesis of GABA, your brain's calming mood regulator and natural valium. Chapter 17 of this book explains how you can increase GABA biosynthesis and intensity naturally and safely, to calm your nerves, moods and anxiety. Drugs can have their place, of course. There are times when it is necessary to take medicines as an emergency measure until you can determine a long-term solution.

PRE-EMPTIVE SELF-MANAGEMENT

When you live in an acidic state of sympathetic dominance, your body's enzymes and neuromessengers do not communicate properly, and numerous metabolic processes, such as digestion, energy production, memory, creativity and cellular repair, slow down as your body becomes sluggish and bogged down. You will probably suffer from gastrointestinal problems such as bloating, gas, constipation and irritable bowel. When your energy production declines, your metabolism slows down as you gather intracellular trash, and you will have less energy, likely gain weight and feel less excitement and passion for life.

Conscious Attention One Day at a Time

As a pre-emptive self-management strategy, direct your energy circuits each day into positive sources that can help you feel filled with health and healing—all this requires is conscious attention. Learn to interpret any early warning, red-alert symptoms as a signal that cortisol and adrenaline are surging and you are losing your vital energy. As a pre-emptive self-management strategy, Caroline Myss, PhD, likes to say, "Let your biography become your biology." You control your nervous system. Don't let it control you.

To have a healthy modern response, you must consciously learn to shift your acidic sympathetic nervous system, run by cortisol and adrenaline rushes, to an alkaline parasympathetic nervous system, run by the hormones DHEA and dopamine.

LAUGHTER AND HUMOR

Throughout your day, feel absolutely free to give loving encouragement to others, which will help both you and them have a successful day. One of the most powerful techniques to free yourself from emotional distress is the practice of laughter and humor. You now know that when you laugh, your body produces lots of the "light," feel-good neuromessengers dopamine, DHEA and beta endorphins, and reduces the "heavy," corrosive stress hormone cortisol. When you lose yourself in laughter, you will find respite from technology and noise for a while, which will uplift your body, mood and state of mind.

"Humorlessness is hostile to health and happiness."
David R. Hawkins, MD, PhD, *Power vs. Force*

BREAKING HABITUAL PATTERNS

It is very easy to get caught in restrictive habits. Therefore, it is extremely helpful to consciously let go or relinquish negative things in your life and create new patterns of thinking and behaving. You become more flexible when you review and purposely adjust old patterns. This brings flexibility to your nervous system also, as your 100 billion brain cells learn to make new associations. You have a positive and negative feedback loop between your nervous system and the choices you make in your life. As you willingly try new lifestyle changes, the neurons in your brain and their enormous communication network become more active, flexible and now open to new perceptions, awareness and choices, which in turn support the growth of many more new neuronal connections. The more connections, the bigger your circuitry board, and the brighter, more enthusiastic, creative and aware you will be.

"There is nothing either good or bad, but thinking makes it so."
William Shakespeare, *Hamlet*

To break out of habitual patterns, try these suggestions:

- turn off your TV and read
- meditate or pray longer
- eat slowly and savor your food
- visit friends and family
- change your exercise program
- listen to different music

SELF-MANAGEMENT WITH MEDITATION MEDICATION

Stop for a moment. Be conscious of your thoughts or breathing. It's obvious: Becoming aware of the moment like this helps you feel more consciously mindful of the moment, more serene, more at peace. And now there is scientific evidence that praying and meditating regularly creates new, positive patterns of thinking, perceiving and behaving, as well as a boost to your immune system. After an eight-week training program of meditation at the University of Wisconsin–Madison, participants showed increased activity in the area of the brain linked to a positive emotional state, contentment, serenity, security and elevated self-esteem. Their immune system also developed 50 percent more antibodies than non-meditators.

Meditation does not mean passivity, but clearer thinking.

Mindful prayer and meditation recognize thoughts and feelings as they surface without acting on them. Try it yourself. Witness the moment without trying to change it. This non-judgmental moment-to-moment awareness is the best self-management technique to create emotional balance and well-being.

THE POWER OF RELEASING SELF-IMPOSED RESTRICTIONS

We are by nature emotional abundance—not limited emotional restriction. We must let go of the emotional baggage that has been getting in the way of doing what we know we want to do, and should be doing, with our life. Change yourself from the inside out. When we change ourselves from the inside out, the change is permanent and we effortlessly glimpse ourselves as we really are—a natural, emotionally unrestricted human being. The only emotional restrictions in our life are all self-imposed. We frequently get emotionally stuck. We can and must release ourselves to experience our full abundance, freedom and pure joy. Our lives will then be full of gratitude and sheer wonder.

Ask yourself, "Am I these limiting feelings, or am I having these feelings?" "But why do I get stuck?" "Am I willing to give myself permission to release my limiting feelings? When?" If you do, you will feel secure as you explore each emerging moment. You will no longer drag yourself through life, going from one emotional battle to another.

There are three possible ways to deal with feelings or emotions:

1. **Express them**. "Let off steam," but the original restriction may still remain. Some feelings of love, respect, kindness, compassion and gratitude are necessary to express daily.
2. **Release them**. Every day, choose to let go of tensions, anxiety and pent-up stress—aaaah!
3. **Suppress them**. They now become lifelong restrictive burdens or limitations to our freedom as we hold on to them and accumulate more and more, until we become emotionally constricted, saturated and heavy.

When we finally release our self-imposed restrictions, we shift our consciousness from one of resistance, internal stress and nerve-racking anxiety to one of emotional and mental freedom to immediately express the pure pleasure of simply being alive in each new, emerging moment for a lifetime. We then can grow into better, loving relationships, self-esteem, more radiant health and the ability to be happy, content, fulfilled and living with genuine purpose, no matter what is going on around us.

When faced with an emotion or feeling that overwhelms or brings a sense of imbalance, step back and observe. Observe the anger, sadness, fear or jealousy. Do not push it away, but do not stay in it. Observe. When you begin to experience some degree of freedom from reacting, feel inside to where the restriction or overwhelming emotion has been coming from. Go to it. Let it take you past the moment of anger, fear, or any negative emotion to the place, in your body, where it really stems from. Perhaps the anger is a deep-seated hurt from the past. Are you really feeling unlovable or abandoned? Take the time to release the restricted emotion by honoring its presence and going within—not looking outward to find your balance, your center. If suddenly, you are awash in painful emotion, such as hatred, negativity or bitterness, see if you can touch and release the awful wounds that give rise to it. Keep coming back to your own feelings—I'm so furious! I have been betrayed! My heart is breaking!—so that rather than staying mired in the accusations, instead you are able to release your own constricting pain.

Practice releasing self-sabotaging feelings—they're like flashing neon signs pointing directly to our own stuck places—during daily "meaningful pauses." Even a little willingness to practice, with a sincere desire to change or transform yourself, will improve your life experience for a lifetime, and benefit the entire world as global wellness. Remember, feelings are only feelings; feelings are not who you really are. You can choose to change your perceptions and feelings, to free yourself to perceive what is actually here. You can then act, or refrain from acting, according to your new perceptions and feelings.

THE ROADMAP TO EMERGING HAPPINESS THROUGH THE POWER OF RELEASING

Self-Imposed Feelings

Abandonment
Apathy
Anger
Anxiety
Arrogance
Belligerence
Boredom
Defiance
Evasiveness
Embarrassment
Envy
Failure
Forgotten
Fear
Laziness
Needing approval
Needing acknowledgment
Humiliated
Hurt
Insecure
Judgmental
Lonely
Proud
Prejudiced
Ruthless
Separation
Unforgiving
Worthless
Sorry

Meaningful Action

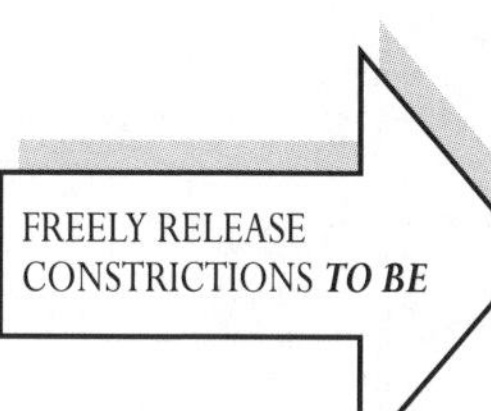

Freedom to Be Natural

Abundant
Accepted
Alive
Boundless
Centered
Content
Fulfilled
Grateful
Happy
Hopeful
Humble
Joyful
Kind
Loving
Peaceful
Pure
Purposeful
Radiant
Spontaneous
Secure
Strong
Successful
Visionary
Whole

As you practice releasing, you will notice that your life is less stressful, less anxious and even your suffering and pain will lessen. Let go once and for all of the emotional restrictions and limiting feelings you have put on yourself. You can!

Do all or most of these recommendations daily. With willpower, you will find they provide you with the strong foundations for a great day. Be healthy. Be happy.

4

WHAT SIGNALS ARE YOU SENDING TO YOUR BODY?

The quality of the food you eat each day is perhaps the most significant factor that determines if you have a great day or not. Your food choices also affect your genes. A fact: What you eat can either help prevent cancer and degenerative disease or actually cause it. Your food choices can contain either body-ready nutrients or body-unrecognizable chemicals. A 1995 survey conducted by the American Institute for Cancer Research highlights this point.

Eighty-six percent of people in the survey thought that genes cause cancer. According to leading researchers, however, only about *10 to 15 percent* of cancers are genetic in origin—*85 to 90 percent* are caused by a combination of diet and environmental and lifestyle factors.

> "One would think we live in precarious times, when lemonade is made from artificial flavors—but—furniture polish is made from real lemons."
>
> Paul Newman

THE ONLY RULE I REQUEST YOU FOLLOW

Only eat cell-friendly foods that will love you back.

Richard Weindruch, PhD, of the University of Wisconsin has conducted research into how genes are affected by dietary change.

This is exactly what my father, Papa Joe, did—he started to use food as medicine.

The results were published in *Scientific American* in 1996. His research, "Nutrient Modulation of Gene Expression," illustrates that by simply reducing the number of total calories eaten, the lifespan of a mouse could be prolonged by 40 percent. In human terms, that would translate into extending the predicted lifespan from today's average of 78.1 years to a healthy age of 95.

REMEMBER THIS IRREFUTABLE FACT

Dr. Weindruch discovered that there are 6,347 genes in a typical mouse. He discovered that during normal aging, when mice could eat as much as they wanted, 5 percent of the mouse's genes underwent an increase in activity and 5 percent decreased. Are you surprised to learn that the 5 percent that rose in activity were stress genes, and the 5 percent that fell were energy genes?

This is what I see daily in those who seek me out for advice. They are fatigued, depressed and stressed. They describe having weak immune systems, memory loss, chronic pain, arthritis and a foggy mind. Until I ask, most have not realized how food and diet have caused many of their symptoms.

In Dr. Weindruch's study, the mice that ate all they wanted experienced far more stress and less energy—and lived on average for 34 months.

The opposite was true among mice that ate less. They maintained their youthful energy, vitality and appearance even as they aged—and lived on average for 65 months.

Roy Walford, MD, a professor of pathology at UCLA medical school, conducted similar research on larger animals, such as monkeys, and even humans. Dr. Walford's research suggests that with a high-nutrient but low-calorie diet a person theoretically can live for approximately 120 years without a severe decline in quality of life.

All of this research points out that you are constantly speaking to your genes, and the words, sentences and instructions are the foods you eat. Moment to moment, your body is buzzing with signals it gets from your food choices. They are transmitted as part of the vast intelligent network that links your mind-body-mood-spirit energy regulators.

FOOD AS MEDICINE

The various elements in food send decisive messages of health or illness to your genes. Most surprising, whether you know it or not, hear it or not, your genes are talking back. You have 100 trillion vibrant dancing cells that send chemical messengers to communicate with each other all over your body. This is the science of intercellular communication, the optimal functioning of which is vitally crucial to your total health, well-being and vibrant energy.

If you are in tune with your body you can hear your 100 trillion dancing cells sending a message, as a signal, like one of these:

1. **Good-Food Day Message**: "Thank you for eating smart, healthy food—it is easy to produce energy galore and there are enough nutrients left so we can fight off this virus that wants to cause a flu bug to gallop from cell to cell. Oh! We just found all the nutrients to synthesize lots of brain messengers called dopamine and serotonin so your brain will be brilliant today and your mood wonderful."

2. **Bad-Food Day Message**: "What are you doing to us by eating dangerously unhealthy food? We are your faithful cells, dedicated to working 24 hours a day, seven days a week, twelve months a year to make you healthy, happy and disease-free. Why are you feeding us with low-grade fuel that causes us to be dysfunctional? We're not feeling well and can't function well, so we have to put

> your body into the *alarm state*, hit the stress button hard, sound the alarms and pump out lots of cortisol and adrenaline, and shut down the energy supply to the brain, the muscles, the eyes, the heart, the skin and the hair. Give us all you've got at each cellular and subcellular level or we won't make it. The addition or omission of a single nutrient in your diet can make or break our energy, attention span, learning and mood."

If you do not feed your body healthy, energy-producing foods, you sacrifice your cells' ability for high-fidelity intercellular communication and your entire body and mind's optimum functioning quickly spirals downward at ever-increasing speeds. When people tell me they experience many debilitating headaches, I ask them to pay strict attention to the continuous communication between their body and their brain. Their headaches are caused by stress, tension and poor digestion.

In his book *Journey into Healing*, Deepak Chopra writes:

> "The body is not a frozen sculpture. It is a river of information—a flowing organism empowered by millions of years of intelligence. Every second of our existence we are creating a new body."

Your food choices dictate the quality of your intercellular communicators and can keep your body and brain in healthy dynamic balance—one day at a time—or lead to communication breakdowns, garbled messages, aborted messages, decay and disease. It's your call! It all depends on how your genes and cells respond to the nutrients they receive from the food you eat. How well you eat tells your cells and genes what type of body and brain you want to have for the rest of your life. Every minute 200 million new cells are renewed and re-energized in your body. That is a total of 300 billion new cells a day. The quality of the food you eat directly influences the developmental efficiency, revitalization, rejuvenation and network communication functioning of each and every one of your cells. Choose wisely!

WHEN ENOUGH IS ENOUGH

I believe very strongly that there is a connection between our fast-paced, fraction-of-a-second world and the rising prevalence of disease today. Let's face it, life moves at such a greater pace than ever before, and most people's nervous systems cannot handle the overload.

Food was, and still is, the original and best medicine.

Back in 1906, disease was deep down and slow. Today, disease, like our multi-tasking, fast-paced, nanosecond society, is characterized by lightning speed.

We ourselves have *upregulated cell overgrowth,* which we call:

- fibromyalgia
- chronic fatigue
- obesity
- diabetes
- memory loss, Alzheimer's, Parkinson's

We ourselves have *under-regulated cell growth,* which we call:

- cancer
- heart disease
- cardiovascular disease
- high blood pressure
- stroke

There is hard scientific proof of a relationship between under-regulated cell growth and upregulated cell overgrowth. As an example, the risk factors for colon cancer are excessive consumption of red meat; low intake of fiber or water in the diet; stress; obesity; and lack of exercise.

"Becoming so productive has given us a new deficiency disease—a severe deficiency of quality free time for ourselves."

Dharma Singh Khalsa, MD

High-frequency stress foods are the processed foods—such as white sugar, high-fructose corn syrup, excessive red meat, fried foods, refined processed foods, excessive alcohol and caffeine—that cause excessive alarm reactions in your body day after day after day. They accumulate damage and can disturb the functioning of susceptible young brains. Essentially, you have the same body chemistry and brain functioning your biological ancestors had two thousand years ago.

We have become used to instant money, instant news, instant communication, instant war, instant stress, instant fear and instant gratification. We have cell phones, cell phone cameras, cell phone television, land phones, pagers, electronic mail and hand-held palm computers. Technology says that this helps us to be more productive!

"NO TIME LEFT FOR..."

Randy Bachman and the Guess Who sang this famous lyric.

Processed, refined foods look good, smell good and taste good, but they have no or, at best, few nutrients. In a fast-paced society your genes receive a hurry-up signal and they obey by speeding up. After all, they are programmed to be faithful. These foods cause an artificial signal and an artificial stimulation to be relayed to your genes and 100 trillion cells. Unfortunately, the only thing really speeding up is your "wear-and-tear," the development of extremely detrimental stress, excessive fatigue, a foggy mind and mangled cell architecture.

Eating healthy foods modulates your genes and cells that regulate the production, as well as the quality and quantity, of your daily energy supply. As a result, you can eat to both prevent and reverse memory and brainpower loss and to increase your well-being, dynamic energy and good moods.

TWELVE SIGNS YOUR CELLS ARE RECEIVING NEGATIVE ALARM SIGNALS AND FLAWED COMMUNICATION FROM UNHEALTHY FOODS

Typical Symptoms	Communication Breakdown
1. foggy mind	glucagon imbalance, not enough protein
2. depression	neurotransmitter dysfunction of serotonin
3. headaches	increase in emotional overload and too many toxic chemicals
4. drop-dead fatigue	poor-quality sleep or a severe sleep debt
5. chronic fatigue	poorly regulated daily detox
6. fibromyalgia	impaired liver, storage of toxic waste
7. attention deficit disorder (ADD)	impaired neurotransmitters
8. obesity	too many calories, insulin imbalance
9. frequent colds and flu	chemicals shutting down immune defenses
10. cancer	overgrowth of dysfunctional acidic cells
11. bad hair or skin days	overly acidic cells
12. stiff, sore muscles and joints	increased level of inflammatory proteins

Adapted from *Improving Intracellular Communication in Managing Chronic Illness* by Jeffrey S. Bland, PhD.

THE TEN NEGATIVE-ALARM FOODS MOST IMPORTANT TO AVOID

Alarm Food	Why
1. donuts	- fried, full of sugar and white flour - can be 35%–40% trans fats - one donut can be 250 calories
2. soft drinks, sodas, pop	- one can of pop has 10 teaspoons of sugar, 150 calories and is loaded with artificial food colours and sulphites - the diet versions have problematic aspartame or sucralose
3. French fries and commercially fried foods	- loaded with trans fats and cell-destructive acrylamide fats -cooked in vegetable oils that cause free radicals
4. corn, potato and tortilla chips	- loaded with trans fats and acrylamides
5. fried non-fish seafood	- commercially frozen fried shrimp, clams and oysters contain trans fats and acrylamides
6. peanuts that are not organic	- commonly contaminated with aflatoxin, a nasty mold
7. sugar (sugar cane and sugar beets)	- fuels obesity - feeds cancer cells - is addictive - fuels ADHD and hyperactivity
8. corn syrup and high-fructose corn syrup	- genetically modified - contains fungi
9. artificially flavored drinks	- elevate insulin levels - contain artificial colours
10. chocolate-flavored commercial milk	- mostly sugar that raises insulin levels

IMPORTANT NOTE: You can eat, in moderation, organic chocolate that is 70 percent cocoa.

SUGAR SENDS ALARM SIGNALS TO YOUR CELLS THAT CAUSE DAILY ENERGY CRISES AND CANCER

Can you imagine the landscape inside your brain, organs and cells as they try to function naturally on a steady supply of processed foods, sugar and chemicals that are difficult to incorporate into your body's biological functions, and were never meant to be part of the original genetic makeup? Pure mayhem—an energy crisis—a sure recipe for exhaustion, chronic illness and mood decline from starving, confused, nutrient-deprived cells in your body and mind.

OUR BRAINS LIKE LITTLE SPURTS OF GLUCOSE SIGNALS FROM FOOD

When we start our car, we need "little hits" or spurts of gasoline to start it. If we flood the motor with "big hits" or big spurts of gasoline, the surging tide of fuel overwhelms the system like a tidal wave, flooding the "on-off" switch, jamming it into "off." We need a maximum of 1 teaspoon or 5 grams of glucose every 3 to 4 hours to give our bodies and brains constant little spurts of sugar as fuel in our bloodstreams. We get this from eating fruits in moderation, vegetables, salads, herbs, sea vegetables and "green drinks." Eat just one average-sized commercial cinnamon bun and you get an overpowering spurt of *12 teaspoons of sugar*, guaranteed to cause hormonal havoc by flooding and jamming your little energy engines into "off." Within 1 hour of eating a sweet treat, surging blood glucose signals insulin levels to spike, causing your physical, emotional and mental performance to decline in an ever-increasing downward spiral. Elevated insulin levels also cause further cravings.

Sugar, sweet treats, alcohol (a carbohydrate) and stimulants are ultimately counterproductive to your physical and emotional well-being. They initially stimulate, but soon begin to exhaust and play havoc with your healthy stability by sending negative, disruptive mind-body signals.

Sugar has always been available in natural sources from fruit, with its slow-releasing fructose balanced by a fiber content that gives our bodies small, constant spurts of glucose, the primary fuel in our bloodstream.

Terry Grossman, MD, an anti-aging physician and co-author of *Fantastic Voyage*, states, "The two chemicals that will age you quicker than anything else are cortisol, a by-product of stress, and elevated insulin, which peaks with sugar consumption." Sugar promotes growth of a broad variety of pathological cells, including the yeast candida albicans and fungal infections. Sugar, a "naked carbohydrate," was introduced to North America by Christopher Columbus in 1493. It has many names, most of which end in -ose, e.g., fructose, glucose, maltose and sucrose. Foods that are almost completely sugar are amasake, honey, maple syrup, molasses and high-fructose corn syrup. Do not use suspect, manufactured fructose added as a sweetener to foods, even healthy foods, since it may appear to support the initiation of cancer.

The number one alarming epidemic for those aged twelve to thirty-four is *type II diabetes*, which is generally caused by a generation swept away by processed foods and everything sweet, which have severe consequences for the brain.

Diabetics age 30 percent faster than the average person, suffer from many more debilitating chronic diseases and accelerated aging so they die far too soon—generally in pain—and are vulnerable to arterial damage, cancer, cardiovascular disease, strokes, loss of critical brainpower and memory, and possibly Alzheimer's disease.

Famed biochemist Dr. Lester Packer at the University of California, Berkeley says, "We can't live without glucose, but over-consumption is extremely toxic." A very little is good—a lot is sweet and deadly.

SUGAR IS LINKED TO CANCER AND DEATH RISK

Findings from the Korean Cancer Prevention Study, published in the January 12, 2005, issue of the *Journal of the American Medical Association*, finally revealed a direct association between elevated blood sugar levels and diabetes and the risk of developing and dying from cancer.

Tumors are primarily obligate glucose (sugar) metabolizers, meaning they require sugar for survival. Even though the brain normally uses high amounts of glucose, a hepatoma (a tumor of the liver), as an example, consumes roughly as much glucose as the brain.

Many North Americans continuously satisfy cancer's appetite by ingesting as much as 295 pounds of sugar a year. Nobel Laureate Otto Warburg, PhD, discovered in 1955 that cancer cells use glucose for fuel. But glucose accomplishes another strategic maneuvre that favors cancer growth: it immobilizes and depresses the abilities of the immune system.

A lifestyle and diet that eliminates all sugars deprives cancer of its primary energy supply and boosts the reliability of the immune system.

SUGAR WINS THE TRIPLE CROWN

The dangers of sugar are finally being ingrained into our collective consciousness. Sugar does its silent but deadly work in three ways: (1) it quickly boosts blood sugar levels, which (2) increases insulin and causes conglomerations of sugar to bind or stick to a protein molecule in a process called glycation. This gums up your critical communication pathways, causing inflammation, free-radical damage to your cells and dramatically accelerates the aging process, which (3) creates a free-radical factory called advanced glycation end-products (AGEs).

AGEs storm and bombard collagen fibers in your skin, causing them to stick together so that the fibers cross-link, stiffen, lose their elasticity or "snap" and cause deep facial wrinkles. Once the proteins are glycated, they continuously generate free radicals that specifically activate the pro-inflammatory peptides TNF-a and NF-kappa B to levels that cause brain cells, communication networks and neuromessengers to degenerate, leading to dementia and Alzheimer's disease. Age spots on your skin indicate formation of AGEs, as does a mental decline in your memory, creativity or motivation. Cataracts in the lens of the eye are another example. Sure makes the bowl of ice cream, the chocolate cake, the piece of pie, cheesecake, cookie or cinnamon bun a lot less appetizing, doesn't it?

TEST YOUR BLOOD SUGAR AND INSULIN LEVELS

Hyperinsulinemia (excess insulin in the blood from excess sugar) has been implicated as a major risk factor in Alzheimer's, heart attacks, diabetes, stroke and cancer. Canadian researcher J.P. Despres and others reported in the *New England Journal of Medicine* that consistently elevated insulin levels is the second leading risk factor for heart attack (male gender is first). They emphasize that an acceptable insulin benchmark level is 5; one over 12 doubles the risk of heart attack, and a level over 15 triples the risk. Have a physician measure and interpret the glucose and insulin levels in your bloodstream.

- A **Fasting Glucose Test** measures the fasting blood sugar level. New optimal levels are 60–80. Results of 80–99 are pre-diabetic and levels exceeding 100 suggest insulin resistance or overt type II diabetes.
- A **Two-Hour Glucose Tolerance Test** challenges a fasting patient with seventy-five grams of sugar in a sweet drink, measuring blood glucose one and two hours later. This test is too insensitive for detecting insulin resistance.
- A **Glucose-Insulin Tolerance Test** is more accurate than the fasting test since both glucose and insulin levels are measured, even in the absence of elevated blood sugar, showing pancreas problems long before the blood sugar rises.
- An **Insulin Challenge Test** is the best diagnostic test for measuring insulin resistance. Unfortunately, it is expensive and involves an intravenous line and the patient must be monitored continuously.
- A **Fasting Insulin and HOMA-IR** fasting serum insulin is used as an index of insulin sensitivity and resistance. Insulin resistance, estimated by homeostasis model assessment (HOMA-IR), has been shown to increase accuracy over traditional tests. HOMA-IR is determined by multiplying the fasting blood glucose level by 10 and then dividing it by 22.5. The lower the number, the better.

OPTIMAL FASTING GLUCOSE AND INSULIN LEVELS

	Optimal Level	Acceptable	High Risk	Normal
fasting insulin	2–3	under 5	over 10	6–25
fasting glucose	60–80	60–99	over 100	60–99

A GOOD ALTERNATIVE SWEETENER

Stevia is an herbal sweetener with natural, medicinal qualities. No negative effects have been discovered, but many health benefits have been observed: It lowers blood sugar in diabetics, and regulates blood sugar levels in non-diabetics. I personally use stevia. Numerous studies have been performed in Japan and in the United States on stevia's effect on cell function, cell membranes, enzyme systems and cancer, and no negative effects have been discovered. Stevia has been valued for its medicinal abilities and natural sweetness in South America, especially Paraguay, for fifteen hundred years.

HEALING MIND-BODY SIGNALS

The relationship between your emotions and your health is turning out to be more interesting and more important than most researchers imagined. Alienation, anxiety, obsessiveness and helplessness are not just feelings. Neither are love, faith, hope and optimism. These are all physiological states that affect your health and well-being as much as healthy food or physical fitness. Your brain, as the source of such states, offers a potential gateway to countless other organs, tissues and cells—from your intestines and immune system to your heart and blood vessels. Researchers have mapped pathways linking mental states to medical ones. Our modern day challenge is to learn how to travel them wisely, at will. The oldest and most proven form of mind-body medicine is sincere prayer.

According to a recent survey, nearly 50 percent of all North Americans use mind-body interventions, such as deep breathing, progressive muscle relaxation, hatha yoga, Tai Chi, acupuncture, guided imagery, mindfulness, meditation or prayer.

THE STRESS RESPONSE

Physiologists recognize that when confronted by a threat—physical or emotional—your body responds with an automatic rise in heart rate, blood pressure, breathing rate, alarm alert and muscle tension. This ancient stress response involves hormones and chemical messengers that buzz through your communication network in small bursts, but if they are released in exaggerated bursts, they initiate everything from tension headaches, migraines, indigestion and constipation to heart attacks. Chronic stress from low-level constant emotional upsets can disrupt your digestive system, interfere with fertility, shut down your immune system or libido, worsen symptoms of menopause and leave you exhausted, collapsing in a heap.

SOOTHING EMOTIONS SIGNAL GOOD HEALTH

Mounting evidence suggests that many soothing emotional experiences can greatly improve your physical health. In the 1970s Dr. Hans Selye started to chart the ill-health effects of hopelessness and hostility and gained unprecedented insight into the mind's power to heal.

> Stress-related illness often defies conventional high-tech medications and procedures.

Researchers used PET scans to compare the brains of Parkinson's sufferers who got placebo intervention with those who got active intervention. As expected, the active intervention caused dopamine, the neurotransmitter circuitry that people with Parkinson's lack, to rise. But those who improved equally in the placebo intervention experienced the same positive dopamine boost.

Now Harvard researchers suggest that the "relaxation response," which comes from deep breathing, meditation or prayer, helps to counter the physical effects of chronic stress. Meanwhile, at Duke University, researchers have found that religious observances are associated with lower rates of all illness and hospitalization. Furthermore, in studies of HIV-positive people, UCLA researchers have found that relentless optimism is associated with stronger immune-cell function.

GOING BEYOND INSPECTIONS AND INJECTIONS

Mind-body techniques can improve anyone's quality of life. Mind-body medicine offers a saner starting point than high-tech medications and procedures. Stress-related illness often defies conventional remedies. Prescription medication and high-tech procedures are an incomplete model of care. Integrating conventional care with complementary and alternative mind-body therapies is immeasurably more friendly, has a more human touch, and involves sympathy, individualized care and friendly communication. Health care providers and patients now become allies in an effort to sustain perseverance and hope in order to find meaning and transformation in suffering.

The medical journal *Lancet* quotes Dr. Salim Yusuf, of McMaster University in Ontario, in a survey of heart attack sufferers: "Stress was comparable to risk factors like hypertension and abdominal obesity. That's much greater than we thought before."

We now believe that your body produces more nitric oxide when deeply relaxed, with no panic or red alerts. Nitric oxide is a molecule that is counter-regulatory, or an antidote, to exaggerated surges of potentially toxic stress hormones like cortisol and adrenaline because it raises the level of beneficial calming hormones and neurotransmitters like gamma amino butyric acid (GABA), DHEA and dopamine. Only five years ago, psychologists in the scientific community told me that this was a lot of mystical mumbo jumbo, but now they're saying that we have to start paying attention.

WAYS TO REDUCE COUNTERPRODUCTIVE RED-ALERT STRESS SIGNALS

Meditation is an ancient practice that elicits a relaxation response to balance out the unavoidable stress responses of daily modern living. Sit quietly in a chair and turn off all radios, televisions, pagers and computers. First, close your eyes and relax your muscles progressively from your feet to your calves, thighs, hips, abdomen, chest, back, shoulders, neck, face and head. Second, choose a short phrase or prayer that is rooted in your belief system, such as "peace," "I am love," "Jesus, guide me," "om," "the Lord is my shepherd," "om mani padme hum," or "God is great." Breathe in your mantra while saying it in your mind and breathe it out slowly and deeply. Sit for 10, 20 or 30 minutes, but even 5 minutes can leave you calm, refreshed and connected.

Deep breathing starts by inhaling slowly and exhaling deeply so your belly expands and contracts. Picture yourself oxygenating all your deep tissues and cells while exhaling physical and emotional toxic trash. Practice for 5, 10 or 15 minutes each morning and again each evening.

Mindfulness has its essence in paying close attention to the moment and your thoughts as well as your body's physical sensations. The guiding principle is to be present moment to moment, and to be aware of what's happening, but without critique or judgment.

Forgive and let live is part of human nature, and appears to favor not just your spiritual well-being, but your physical health as well. It even has its own foundation—A Campaign for Forgiveness Research—and is one of the hottest fields of research in clinical psychology today. "Forgiveness is a healthful alternative to anger and vengeance," states philosopher Mark Huthmacher.

Forgiveness does not require you to forego justice.

Forgiveness works in at least two ways. One is by reducing the debilitating stress of the state of unforgiveness—a mixture of anger, hostility, bitterness, resentment, hatred and fear of being humiliated again. These emotional instabilities increase blood pressure, cause your hair to fall out and spark hormonal changes that are linked to immune suppression, cardiovascular disease, stroke and impaired memory or neurological function. The other benefit of forgiveness is that it keeps strong social networks of family, friends and neighbors together, since keeping grudges will alienate some relationships.

Forgiveness is the best pre-emptive, self-management technique to ensure you have a peaceful, serene, tranquil and happy heart.

Forgiveness turns out to be surprisingly complex. Dr. Dean Ornish says, "When I talk about forgiveness, I mean letting go of your own suffering." "Forgiveness is a process, not a moment," writes Dr. Edward M. Hallowell, a Harvard psychiatrist and author of *Dare to Forgive*. Forgiveness, he emphasizes, has to be cultivated; it goes against a natural human tendency to seek revenge. For this reason he recommends doing it with the help of friends or a therapist or through prayer. The message is the same whether it's spliced into the language of Christian charity, Buddhist mindfulness, the wisdom of Confucius or clinical psychology. Says Dr. Hallowell, "If you devote your life to seeking revenge, first dig two graves."

PEAK PERFORMANCE SIGNALS

Jarome Iginla is one of the world's best hockey players and he is presently captain of the Calgary Flames hockey club. He had just completed his rookie year in the NHL and won the prestigious honor of Rookie of the Year when he came to see me.

Jarome told me that he had to stay energized, to keep moving to be at the top of his game. He said, "The season is long and there is extensive travel with high expectations that you play well every night." I explained that he had to send revitalizing signals to his cells daily.

I designed an energizing, cell-friendly nutritional program for Jarome and I highly recommended that he constantly use positive self-images of being energized and playing at peak performance. He was open and receptive to making changes in his lifestyle. He has such a positive attitude and outlook.

Job well done, Jarome!

Protect your faithful, hard-working cells. Give them natural, cell-friendly, healthy emotions, lifestyle and food so they can have the highest quality fuel possible and give you many years of enormous energy, wellness and well-being. Do it one day at a time. That is all I ask of you. Remember, one great day *equals* one great life.

5

TURN OFF YOUR ENERGY ZAPPERS

TIRED OF FEELING TIRED?

Did you get up this morning feeling wide awake, bursting with energy to take on the day, or did you moan, slap the snooze button, groan and wonder how you would have the energy to do everything you needed to do?

If you have been suffering from roller coaster energy blackouts, chances are that you need an overhaul. Here are the ten energy-zapping errors that you might be making and how to resolve them.

1 Drinking Like a Camel

More than half of your body is made up of good old H_20, which lubricates cells. Camels can lose up to 30 percent of their body water and still perform at optimum, but human peak performance starts to deteriorate when even a small amount is lost. Crystal Andrus, author of *Simply... Woman!* states that "with a loss of just 5 percent of your body fluid, immediate symptoms appear: headache, confusion, fatigue, forgetfulness and an elevated heart rate." Losses of less than 5 percent can result in a lack of energy, mental fog, weakness, thirst, dry skin and mouth, and dark, strong-smelling, concentrated urine.

Staying hydrated is a simple strategy to fight fatigue. Drink six to eight full glasses of cell-friendly water throughout the day.

2 Going Too Long Without Eating

Your body needs to be fed fuel at least every 4 hours, even though you have conditioned yourself to go for 6, 7 or 8 hours without eating. Dr. Joey Shulman, in her book *Winning the Food Fight*, warns that "regardless of what you eat, don't go more than four hours without eating or you're going to feel drained."

3 Skipping Breakfast

Eat breakfast every morning because you have just gone through an eight-hour fast while sleeping. Have the protein power shake I designed for Olympic athletes because it is hormonally balanced and will keep your 100 trillion little molecular motors, your faithful cells, humming with peak performance.

JUMP START YOUR DAY WITH MY ONE-MINUTE BREAKFAST

- 8 oz of water, unsweetened rice milk, soy milk, hemp milk or skim organic milk
- 2–4 heaping tablespoons of organic, low-fat plain soy or dairy yogurt
- 2 scoops of high-alpha whey protein isolate powder
- 1 full cup of any fresh or frozen berry such as blueberries, blackberries or raspberries
- 2 tablespoons of both organic flax seeds and sesame seeds, 30 grams each, ground fresh in a coffee grinder for the lignan fibers and the short-chain omega-3 fats
- ½ teaspoon of organic borage oil—for the bioactive omega-6 fatty acid, gamma linolenic acid, or a 500 milligram capsule of evening primrose oil for omega-6 fatty acids

Blend all ingredients in a blender for 10 seconds on low so that you do not denature the whey protein isolate powder.

- 1 softgel of enteric-coated concentrate wild, triple fish oil so that you get 300 percent better absorption and no "fishy" aftertaste. Use fish oils rich in "mood smart" EPA and "brain smart" DHA, supercritical fats that your brain needs daily for good moods, enhanced memory and increased brainpower.

4 Not Being Alkaline and Energized

You must get alkaline to get energized. Your 100 trillion little cells produce enormous energy each day and the by-product of cellular metabolism is acids. As you read these words, your body is generating acid, but don't worry because it's really just a by-product of natural cell function. The acids your body produces are relatively weak and usually do not cause any problems. Your lungs eliminate them every time you exhale.

Sometimes, however, your body gets signals to produce excess acid. This can happen when you eat too many proteins, grains, sugars or dairy products. It can also be caused by strenuous exercise or excess acute stress. This acid is excreted in your urine, and is a signal that your body chemistry is not in balance. In fact, the acid level in your body may be a major factor in determining your level of health.

What happens when your body is too acidic? Researchers believe that your health can be impaired as a result of the following effects:

- free radical oxidation occurs with greater ease, while antioxidant activity is impaired
- vitamins and minerals from foods or supplements are not absorbed well
- friendly bacteria in the small intestines die and the immune system is impaired
- connective tissue becomes weakened, causing skin and hair to lose their tone
- sleep patterns are disturbed
- colds, infections, headaches and flu become more common
- physical and mental energy is depleted, affecting stamina, alertness and moods

You must eat more fresh, colorful, in-season salads, vegetables, herbs, sea vegetables, vegetable juices and fruit.

For the quickest way to become favorably alkaline and get energized, do what I do every morning—use an extra-energy "green drink" supplement.

The second quickest way to relieve acidity in your system is to breathe slowly and deeply several times a day to force alkalinizing fresh oxygen into your deep tissues and to force out stale, acidic carbon dioxide. Oxygen is the first and foremost of all cell-friendly nutrients.

5 Following One-Size-Fits-All Nutrient Plans

When it comes to energy, designing a program to keep you at peak performance is critical. You may need to modify certain foods depending on the time of year and your personal needs. Liz Applegate, PhD, in *Eat Smart Play Hard*, emphasizes that "When you tailor your nutrient needs, you begin to address your personal lifestyle and your eating patterns." You need to ask, "What is it I'm going to give up? What will allow me to stay on this eating pattern so I don't feel I'm begrudging myself?" This is tailoring for success.

6 Dropping Calories Too Low

Take your ideal weight and multiply by 12 and that is the *minimum* number of calories you require each day. I weigh 170 pounds so 170 × 12 = 2,040 calories daily. A diet too low in calories will zap you of energy.

Dieting can also result in a lack of essential vitamins, minerals, antioxidants and phytonutrients, which will reduce your energy level.

7 Not Adjusting Macronutrients

Your body is like a carburetor and you need to fine-tune the mixtures of food you are eating. Your aim is to make your body run at maximum efficiency, which logically will provide maximum energy. With a little attention to detail, you'll be able to pinpoint the combinations that work for you.

Do you need more or less protein? Do you need more or less fat? Do you need more or less low glycemic carbohydrates? Do you need more or less water? Don't completely eliminate carbs, fat or protein from your diet no matter how famous the diet guru is. By the way, fad dieting is dangerous, archaic and downright unhealthy.

Buyer beware, "fat free" does not mean "problem free." Most fat-free foods taste terrible so manufacturers fill them up with notoriously unhealthy sugar, fructose, or high fructose corn syrup that are the real culprits for putting excessive weight on your body. The only low-fat foods I recommend are low-fat, plain, organic yogurt and cottage cheese.

Limit your intake of table salt; processed sodium chloride is as bad for you as any other processed food. Table salt may also contain unnecessary ingredients, such as dextrose, sodium silico, aluminum, sodium and magnesium carbonate, and yellow prussiate of soda, added to table salt to maintain its pure white color. Kosher salt does not contain any of these unnecessary ingredients. Sea salt, in moderation, is salt's natural form and is necessary for good cellular functioning and support, especially for the pituitary, adrenal, kidney, thyroid and pancreas. I personally prefer Celtic sea salt, which has a very high mineral content.

Studies have shown that it takes diligent washing to remove the pesticide residues that are present on fruits and vegetables. For this reason, I recommend that you purchase organically grown foods when possible. Although they may cost a little more, you can feel confident that you and your family are not consuming unnecessary toxins along with your meals. You will also know you are doing your share to reduce the accumulation of toxins in your environment. The potentially higher cost to purchase organic fruits and vegetables does not compare to the price of your health.

The top ten most heavily sprayed foods to purchase organically grown are:

1. lettuce and parsley
2. wheat
3. strawberries
4. green beans
5. celery
6. apples
7. peaches
8. grapes
9. spinach
10. pears

8 Neglecting the Whole Person

Your diet or lifestyle can quickly correct a nutrient or hormonal imbalance, but most energy issues are generally not that simple.

It takes integrated medicine, a holistic approach that balances your four fundamental energy centers: dynamic physical, mental, emotional and spiritual well-being. To overcome fatigue, dragging and stress and improve vitality, you have to look at the whole you and fine-tune your whole lifestyle. For example, depression and stress can lead to exhaustion, lack of alertness and reduced immunity so that you catch more colds or flus.

Don't follow fad diets that promise you will lose 10 pounds in seven days. If you follow an extreme diet, you can kiss your robust vitality and energy goodbye. Modify your program from time to time to fit your specific needs with a positive attitude. As Michael Colgan, PhD, says, "Use your head if you really want to affect your body."

Laugh and smile as much as possible. Laughter reduces stressful cortisol and adrenaline levels by 70 percent and raises your feel good neuromessengers dopamine, DHEA and beta endorphin levels by 40 percent. Smile—it is healthy and allows good moods to soar.

Slow down. The most effective way to tame your jittery nerves and put the brakes on a fast-paced life is to meditate. Herbert Benson, MD, of Harvard Medical School has studied the physiological changes that happen in your body when you meditate. He emphasizes that meditation restores a healthy rhythm to your nervous system by counteracting the fight-or-flight effect of the sympathetic nervous system. When you relax, your parasympathetic nervous system tunes down brain waves from the frazzled beta waves to alert but peaceful and creative alpha waves.

Not Eating Energizing Foods

In my opinion, here's how to get the twelve best energy-boosting foods:

1. Use a natural, "green drink"-based extra energy food supplement containing the amino acids tyrosine, taurine and glycine, as well as vitamins C and B6 and energizing herbs. This is a powerful energy revitalizer that is fast-acting and uplifting to ensure that you are energized for peak performance all day long.

2. Have a powerful, hormone-balancing protein shake for breakfast using whey isolate, hemp or soy protein powders to balance the hormones insulin and glucagon. By balancing insulin and glucagon, you regulate energy all day long.

3. Drink a fresh glass of vegetable juice, such as a combination of carrot, parsley, watercress, cilantro, celery, beet, ginger and a dash of lemon juice.

4. Eat berries, including blueberries, blackberries, raspberries and strawberries.

5. Drink organic green, matcha, oolong, rooibos or peppermint teas.

6. Eat fresh, wild, cold-water salmon, or take a daily supplement with enteric-coated triple fish oil softgels rich in the long-chain omega-3 essential fatty acids "mood-smart" EPA and "brain-smart" DHA.

7. Enjoy zesty, colorful salads and vegetables with sunflower, broccoli, radish, garlic, peas or daikon sprouts. Eat something raw at each of your meals to aid digestion. These foods supply critical fiber to gently sweep your colon clean.

8. Eat fresh, ripe seasonal fruit or melons such as dark-skinned apples, black cherries, mangoes, prunes, watermelon, cantaloupe, papaya, oranges and pink grapefruit.

9. Eat fermented foods such as miso, natto, tempeh, apple cider vinegar or plain, low-fat yogurt, or bitter vegetables like kale, watercress and Swiss chard for good intestinal bacteria to help digest and absorb food nutrients necessary to energize yourself. These foods initiate peristalsis of colon muscles to excrete waste material.

10. Enjoy unsalted, raw seeds such as flax, sesame, sunflower and pumpkin, chewed well, and also unsalted, raw nuts such as almonds, macadamias, Brazil nuts and walnuts.

11. Women's bodies are composed of 65 percent water and men's bodies 68 percent. Water is critical to maintain an anabolic drive and produce optimal energy. Water is the fluid responsible for and involved in regulating every biological process, from synthesizing hormones to ultimate mental acuity. Drink eight to ten eight-ounce

glasses of water daily. Prehydrate—do not wait until you dehydrate. Staying hydrated is a simple strategy to fight fatigue.

12. Surprisingly, organic chocolate that is a minimum of 70 percent cocoa can be considered an energizing food if eaten in moderation about 3:00 p.m. By mid-afternoon your "mood-balancing" hormone seratonin, "good mood" hormone DHEA and neuropeptide beta endorphin levels take a natural dip. If you consume up to one-and-a-half ounces (forty-two grams) of dark, semi-sweet chocolate, which contains only ninety calories, you quickly boost the seratonin, DHEA, and neuropeptide beta endorphin levels so you feel happy, satisfied and content. Amazingly, cancer researchers at Georgetown University recently discovered that the cacao plant (which is the source of chocolate) contains a potent antioxidant called pentamer that increases the activity of cancer-suppressing genes.

10 Getting Inadequate Sleep and Rest

Sleep is not a waste of time. Take time to reflect on your lifestyle. Ask yourself: Is my lifestyle appropriate for my optimal well-being? One of the main reasons most people are exhausted is because they are in sleep deprivation. The National Sleep Foundation encourages adults to get between 7 to 9 hours of sleep each night. If you do not get sufficient sleep, you accumulate a sleep debt that becomes too big to repay, yet the average North American gets fewer than 7 hours of sleep a night and 68 percent are classified as sleep deprived. This resulting sleep deprivation is linked to negative moods, aggressiveness, daytime fatigue, decreased productivity and an increase in both domestic and workplace accident rates.

The Centre for Sleep Study at the University of British Columbia recommends that we go to sleep at the same time each night and wake up at the same time each morning so that our bodies learn a sleeping rhythm. To be able to sleep deeply, you must sleep in a room that is as dark as possible. Receptor cells both in our eyes and on our skin monitor the amount of daylight that is entering the eyes or reaching the skin. If your skin and eyes receive even a small bit of light from illuminated clocks, blinking VCRs, nightlights, or streetlights that come through curtains, your body sends a message that you still need to be alert and attentive. It is only in complete darkness that the body can send a message that everything else is asleep so we do not have to be alert and can naturally fall into a deep sleep. It is only in deep darkness that your pineal gland will synthesize the hormone melatonin, which is responsible for putting us into a deep, rejuvenating sleep. If you do this, you will sleep as nature intended you to.

Most of us don't want to say goodnight to fun and responsibility. The telephone, the Internet, email, eBay and one hundred television channels all rob us of sleep. We have extended the wear-and-tear of our waking day and shortened the restorative dark phase of the circadian cycle through artificial light.

Every night we move further and further from the 9 to 10 hours of sleep that the average adult got in 1920. Each weekday night we get 1 hour and 36 minutes less, on average, than the 8½ hours that sleep experts recommend. Each weekend night we receive 1 full hour less.

By the end of the year, we are short 458 hours—almost three full weeks—of sleep. During an eighty-year lifespan, we fall short an enormous 36,640 hours, or 218 full weeks' worth, of lost sleep. We are the "great unslept," working our way through life on the verge of sleep bankruptcy. Chronic inadequate sleep affects 70 percent of all adults.

What are the consequences of being sleep deprived? The disruption of the natural circadian rhythm our biological ancestors so beautifully adapted to has led to serious consequences for modern humans. In 1940, only 20 percent of North Americans died from a combination of cancer, diabetes, heart disease and stroke. In 2006, nearly 90 percent will die from a combination of cancer, heart disease, stroke and the complications of diabetes. The increase in these degenerative diseases coincides and grafts exactly with our getting less sleep, staying up later because of artificial light, and eating more processed, refined foods.

As you sleep in a deep and regenerative delta state of 3.5 Hz brain waves, your brain is relaxed and open to accept your unconscious dream state. Your brain, at this time, can process new information and purge excess information, leaving you refreshed, renewed and rejuvenated the next day.

6

DOWNSHIFT YOUR TASTE BUDS AND YOUR LIFE

ZESTY NEW TASTE BUDS

Changing from the typical North American diet of processed, sugary, fatty and seductive foods is a healthy change and is certainly easier to follow than you might think.

Too many diets based on moderation—such as limiting yourself to only small amounts of sugar, or one egg yolk every three days, or to no more than 30 percent of calories from fat, or to only 6 ounces of lean meat per day—soon become too time-consuming to calculate and too tedious to follow and tinker with.

Quitting smoking, for most people, is much easier than limiting yourself to one or two cigarettes a day. It is easier to totally avoid less-than-healthy foods like French fries than continually tempt yourself with a few fries every time you eat out. It is easier to have none of the foods you are addicted to than just a few of them. There is no such thing as eating only 1 tablespoon of ice cream or 2 potato chips.

Your number one challenge in downshifting your taste buds with major changes in eating habits is confronting unhealthy, seductive, addictive "food stuff" everywhere. For example, when you first quit smoking, it seems like everyone around you is always smoking. However, these changes soon become second nature, as I have seen over and over again in my twenty-five years of nutritional and lifestyle research.

REMEMBER THIS ONE IRREFUTABLE FACT

"The human central nervous system clearly has an exquisitely sensitive capacity to differentiate between *life-supportive and life-destructive* patterns."

David R. Hawkins, MD, PhD, author of *Power vs. Force*

TWENTY-ONE DAYS TO NEW TASTE BUDS

Your taste buds have a memory of about only twenty-one days. This is an advantage when you downshift your diet. Have you ever switched from whole milk to skim milk? I had my father, Papa Joe, do this as one of his first diet changes or downshifts. At first the lower-fat skim milk seemed excessively watery and just did not taste good to him. But what happened after twenty-one days? Skim milk tasted normal. Whenever he tried whole milk again, it seemed far too thick and fatty. In just twenty-one days Papa Joe's taste preference changed.

"The single most significant change we are witnessing in this Age of Aquarius is how it revolves around experience rather than information."

Dharma Singh Khalsa, MD, *Food as Medicine*

When you try to change or fine-tune your entire diet, you will have many more whole-milk-to-skim-milk experiences to contend with. At first people complain, balk and fuss a bit. I start everyone on a natural, extra-energy "green drink" powder to alkalinize their bodies for an immediate, powerful energy upshift. Within twenty-one days, their taste buds adapt, and the other food adjustments they make become accepted as better than the processed foods they replace. After your taste buds adjust, your desire for the processed, heavy foods will be gone.

A NEW FUTURE BEGINS WITH ONE TURNING POINT

A healthy diet change can work wonders. Linda, for example, was really hooked and seduced by sugar. She was an office worker and got very little exercise. She could control her appetite at work, but every evening after her stressful work day, she wanted ice cream, fancy cheesecakes and fine pastries. Linda was in her early thirties at the time and assumed that her sugar addiction was unconquerable. Her self-esteem was way down, her weight up 40 pounds and her physical health beginning to deteriorate. Her complexion was questionable and her hair had lost its lustre. She complained of constant fatigue.

Linda and her boyfriend, Tim, happened to see a half-hour television program on which I was featured. She decided to purchase one of my books, *The Food Connection*, and follow my recommendations. Her motivation and determination kept her going, and after the initial seven days she had lost 3 pounds, which motivated her to continue. After the full twenty-one-day health experience she had lost 8 pounds of fat, was sleeping soundly and had more energy than she had had in years. She was delighted that her skin was so much clearer and her hair radiant.

Linda was a borderline type II diabetic and checked her morning blood-sugar levels. The turning point for Linda was when after just twenty-one days, her blood-sugar levels dropped from 125 mg/dl to a vibrantly healthy 80 mg/dl (a measure over 125 is considered diabetic). Linda took control of her own life and was free to choose a new and healthy lifestyle.

Linda now says, "I just do not want to return to eating unhealthy foods anymore. I have broken the addiction-seduction attraction. For the first time in ten years, sugary sweet treats do not control me in supermarkets, at convenience stores or even walking past bakeries." She happily states, "I now have a whole new level of wellness and energetic vitality with my new way of eating foods that keeps me fit and healthy." Tim has had great results also.

Remember, it takes twenty-one days to downshift your taste buds back to their natural state of functioning. Hang in there for twenty-one days so you will feel your energy soar. You will soon feel better all day long, all life long.

As they say, the rest is history.

Though we seem to be sleeping,
There is an inner wakefulness
That directs the dream,
And that will eventually startle us back
To the truth of who we are.

Rumi, 12th century Persian mystic poet

Rumi's playful poems encourage us to celebrate the sacredness of every day.

DOWNSHIFT YOUR LIFE

Voluntary simplicity! I like to call it downshifting out of the rat race and upshifting into the human race.

The world around you may be saying:

- do more…
- work harder…
- you gotta be there…
- don't miss this party…
- you need more money…
- you gotta see it, it's a must see TV program…
- you can't live without a big SED flat-panel technology TV…
- it's only three easy payments of $19.95—don't wait—call now…
- this is the ultimate car of your dreams; your life would be great with it…

But, maybe it is time to step back and see the world anew. If you are truly ready to balance your life and free yourself from the *artificial constraints* of our modern world, now may be the time to re-evaluate your life. Come to think of it, seek ways to feel more personally fulfilled every day.

In the business world today, time-management psychologists are teaching appropriate "exit strategies" to countless stressed-out, buzzed-out, good people who want to learn to downshift a wee bit, and take control of their own futures. You could begin by simply doing what my personal assistant, Purna Ma, does—downshift consumer ambitions. She has become a master of finding extremely high-quality clothing at $5 to $10 by shopping at Value Village. My neighbors Elvira and Mark say, "No, we don't need a TV."

Be courageous and creative to live a life that supports your own beliefs.

One recent survey of one thousand adults by the New York-based Families and Work Institute states:

> "Our findings strongly suggest that many employees are reaching a point when increasing work demands simply become too much so that personal and family relations, personal health and the quality of work itself are seriously threatened."

Dr. Wayne W. Dyer, author of *10 Secrets for Success and Inner Peace*, states, "The way to create lasting, life-affirming lifestyle change is through focusing on long-lasting fulfillment, rather than short term fixes."

Many people are now finding practical ways to break free from the work-spend-consumer straitjacket that binds so many. Quietly, but quite radically, many people are learning to simplify their lives so they have more quality time for family, friends, meditation, Pilates, Tai Chi, hatha yoga, exercise, walking in nature, preparing nutritious foods, and more leisurely pursuits to enjoy a richer, happier, more fulfilled life.

"If your life is in harmony...then your life is full and good, but not overcrowded. If it is overcrowded, you are doing more than is right for you, more than is your job to do in the total scheme of things."

Peace Pilgrim

There is growing discontent with our nanosecond, multi-tasking, stressful, money-driven lifestyles. You could begin by simply toning down excessive commitments. You do not need to wait for someone to give you permission. Seize control of your own life and destiny and deliberately change your stressful life to a healthy one.

Check the list below and find the column that best describes your lifestyle right now. Be honest!

WHAT IS YOUR LIFESTYLE?

Ambitious Consumer	Downshifter
– picking up prepared suppers	– preparing healthy meals
– stock market	– farmers' market
– fashion	– comfort
– celebrity culture	– horticulture
– securing capital	– social capital
– bankability	– sustainability
– retain therapy	– aromatherapy
– live to work	– work to live
– fashion magazines	– gardening magazines
– faithful consumer	– faithful citizen
– going to the mall	– going for a walk
– quantity	– quality
– computerized	– socialized
– corporate wellness	– family wellness
– like being served food	– like serving food
– inside information	– insight information
– achieving wealth	– achieving health
– I love restaurant food	– I like home-made food
– too scared to stop	– too tired to keep going
– too busy to be tired	– tired of being tired
Total Score: ________	**Total Score:** ________

If you checked off ten or more boxes in the "Ambitious Consumer" column, read Chapter 3, "One Great Day *Equals* One Great Life" carefully. If you checked off ten or more boxes in the "Downshifter" column, you are on the Path to Phenomenal Health. Don't miss Chapter 13, "Spiritual Insights: Be Inspired."

THE BEGINNING...NOT THE END

A powerful way to loosen the grip of stress from our lives is to go on an immediate media fast. Avoid television, videos, the movies, the daily news, and radios for a day, a week or longer!

I am writing this book by longhand—I have no computer, cell phone, pager, answering machine or microwave. I am writing at my kitchen table as the first soft fire of autumn is glowing in the wood stove. I have learned the art of chopping wood with an axe and have become fairly good at it. It is an art to learn to split logs well.

Living well, being happy and experiencing peace of mind is our birthright and our responsibility to create for ourselves. To make the lifestyle change that you desire, you must be persistent in maintaining a powerful positive attitude. My father was fond of repeating, "Believe and you will succeed."

Deepak Chopra emphasizes that you have eighty thousand ideas and thoughts that enter your subconscious mind daily. Downshifting and clearing your mind is so important as a daily mental exercise. The best form of this exercise is daily prayer, meditation or sitting calmly and quietly, in sheer awe of nature or the night sky.

I have learned some wonderful things and some painful things about myself in the process of downshifting. I have learned that, at any given moment, my thoughts can create a living heaven or a living hell.

I do not know of your personal past losses or failures. I have had many. I do not know your personal pains and challenges. I have had many. I hope I have learned wisely from them and I am grateful for these learning experiences. But what I do know for sure is the power of the human spirit and our infinite potential.

Everyone must downshift differently by varying degrees. We are either a "tiptoer" or a "plunger." Let me share with you the one simple principle I use to downshift. In the third chapter, Nelson Mandela's quote referred to your life as "a garden"; you plant and fertilize your own seeds by everything you do. Every morning when I first meet my image in the mirror, I say, "I love you. What kind of person will you be today? How will you plant your garden, Sam?" You must also ask yourself what kind of person you need to be today to be inspired, and review your day before you go to sleep tonight. Ask yourself this question...then live your answer.

Before you go to sleep at day's end, greet yourself in the mirror. Hold yourself as a precious gift. Ask yourself, "How do I want to live, talk, think, move, feel and love tomorrow?" Your answers, borne out of free choice, will allow you to transform your life from ordinary to remarkable. As Ringo Starr and the Beatles once said, "All you have to do is act naturally."

ACUTE STRESS CAUSES DEPRESSION, STROKES AND HEART ATTACKS

The Japanese have a word for it—*karoshi*, or "death from overwork." But can acute stress on the job really shorten your life?

Finnish researchers decided to find the answer to this question. From 1991 to 1993 Finland experienced an economic meltdown, with unemployment nearly tripling to 17 percent. Those who survived the downsizing had to assume greater workloads. During this period and for seven years afterward, Dr. Jussi Vahtera and psychologist Mika Kivinmaki of the Finnish Institute of Occupational Health in Helsinki followed municipal workers who survived the cutbacks in four towns—from the mayor to nurses, teachers and janitors. Their sobering conclusion appeared in the *British Medical Journal*. Kivimaki puts it bluntly: "The only difference in mortality was in cardiovascular deaths. Those in work units with the most downsizing suffered twice the death rate from heart attack and stroke."

Depression Is More Worrisome Than Smoking or Cholesterol

The American Heart Association journal *Stroke* reports that a research team found that the effect of depression on stroke mortality is greater than smoking or cholesterol. They suggest that a reduction in depressive symptoms in people whose risk for heart disease is above average could significantly reduce future stroke mortality. Depression lowers all of your brain's communication network neuromessengers and, specifically, mood-regulating "messengers" like acetylcholine, GABA, DHEA, dopamine and serotonin, and raises red-alert, destructive mood-regulating cortisol and adrenaline.

In many cases, depressed people who lack key nutrients such as eicosapentaenoic acid (EPA), docosahexaenoic acid (DHA), folic acid and B vitamins respond quite well to supplements to treat depression, especially EPA-rich enteric-coated fish oils like *o3mega+ joy*, rich in EPA essential fatty acids; high-dose folic acid or B9; S-adenosyl-methionine (SAMe); and a sublingual, neuro-supportive form of B12 called methylcobalamin, which help to maintain stable moods.

Today scientists are using high-tech instruments to elucidate the mind-body connections that damage the heart. When you are frightened, your heart begins to pound. When you get angry, your face flushes as your blood pressure rises. Unquestionably, research increasingly shows that if belligerence puts you at risk, a life of quiet regret and guilt does, too. Study after study has now confirmed that factors like social isolation, depression, moodiness and poor marital relations can contribute to heart disease and strokes. Heart-attack survivors who live alone die at twice the rate of those who live with others. When your body responds with a red-alert response to everyday stressors like personality conflicts at work, stalled traffic, a pushy boss, honking horns and looming deadlines, your cardiovascular system suffers. No one is entirely risk free. We all need to calm down and stop obsessing—as Proverbs 17:22 states, a cheerful heart is a good medicine.

THE PARADOX OF OUR AGE

The paradox of our time in history is that we have taller buildings but shorter tempers, wider freeways, but narrower viewpoints. We spend more, but have less, we buy more, but enjoy less. We have bigger houses and smaller families, more conveniences, but less time. We have more degrees but less sense, more knowledge, but less judgment, more experts, yet more problems, more medicine, but less wellness.

We drink too much, smoke too much, spend too recklessly, laugh too little, drive too fast, get too angry, stay up too late, get up too tired, read too little, watch TV too much, and pray too seldom. We have multiplied our possessions, but reduced our values. We talk too much, love too seldom, and hate too often. We've learned how to make a living, but not a life.

We've added years to life not life to years. We've been all the way to the moon and back, but have trouble crossing the street to meet a new neighbor. We conquered outer space but not inner space. We've done larger things, but not better things. We've cleaned up the air, but polluted the soul. We've conquered the atom, but not our prejudice. We write more, but learn less. We plan more, but accomplish less. We've learned to rush, but not to wait. We build more computers to hold more information, to produce more copies than ever, but we communicate less and less.

These are the times of fast foods and slow digestion, big men and small character, steep profits and shallow relationships. These are the days of two incomes but more divorce, fancier houses, but broken homes. These are days of quick trips, disposable diapers, throwaway morality, one night stands, overweight bodies, and pills that do everything from cheer, to quiet, to kill. It is a time when there is much in the showroom window and nothing in the stockroom. A time when technology can bring this letter to you, and a time when you can choose either to share this insight, or to just hit delete.

Remember, spend some time with your loved ones, because they are not going to be around forever. Remember, say a kind word to someone who looks up to you in awe, because that little person soon will grow up and leave your side. Remember, to give a warm hug to the one next to you, because that is the only treasure you can give with your heart and it doesn't cost a cent. Remember, to say, "I love you" to your partner and your loved ones, but most of all, mean it. A kiss and an embrace will mend hurt when it comes from deep inside of you. Remember to hold hands and cherish the moment for someday that person will not be there again.

Give time to love, give time to speak, and give time to share the precious thoughts in your mind. Life is not measured by the number of breaths we take, but by the moments that take our breath away.

Dr. Bob Moorehead, *Words Aptly Spoken*

7

FOOD AS MEDICINE—CELL-FRIENDLY EATING

THE SCIENTIFIC BASIS TO FOOD AS MEDICINE

The renowned Michael Fossel, MD, PhD, Clinical Professor of Medicine at Michigan State University, said these revolutionary words to me: "Use food as medicine—eat a cell-friendly diet." At that time I was a well-recognized Nutritional Lifestyle Researcher. I had started a successful research company in the United States called Advanced Nutritional Research (ANR), which specialized in making cutting-edge supplements for orthomolecular physicians, and I had been fortunate to have worked with the two-time Nobel Prize winner Linus Pauling, PhD, Dr. Zoltan Rona, MD, Dr. Robert Atkins, Dr. Julian Whitaker, Dr. Lester Packer, Dr. Karlis Ullis of UCLA, the renowned psychiatrist Dr. Abram Hoffer, and the father of the free radical theory, Dr. Denham Harman, MD, PhD, of the University of Nebraska.

Dr. Fossel's words struck me deeply and the echo kept penetrating my imagination—eat a cell-friendly diet and use food as medicine.

The scientific basis to Integrative Medicine is simple: balance your mind-body-mood-spiritual energy centers simultaneously.

When I followed my cells back through their genetic lineage, I quickly realized that I was part of a line of cells that were thousands of years old. I didn't teach them how to function, or repair, or renew or revitalize. They already knew how, as they had been designed in the Divine Blueprint.

MASTERING THIS BOOK—FOR A LIFETIME

This book is about the practical scientific breakthroughs you can use today to keep each of your 100 trillion cells efficiently repairing, restoring and rejuvenating so you can immediately boost your radiant vitality, wellness and mental performance from ordinary to remarkable in twenty-one days. I want you to experience optimum energy all day long, all life long. Energy is the currency of life. Peak energy production, whether at twenty-four or eighty-four years of age, means the very same thing—peak performance.

OLD MYTH

You are born with a limited, predetermined genetic inheritance—a limited machine, at best a limited computer, slowly wearing out. Not true!

NEW REALITY

Pioneering research is happening at a whirlwind pace. You can boost and then maintain your energetic vitality and mental performance—all life long—through diet, lifestyle changes, therapeutic supplements, and mental as well as physical activity.

The various components in food send decisive messages of health or illness to your genes. Your genes talk back to you. Your 100 trillion dancing cells send chemical messages to communicate balance all over your body. Eat a cell-friendly diet to achieve good intercellular communication networks.

I have seen several cancer patients recover completely after considered to be incurable. It is not a miracle. We need not battle against death, we need the will to win. This is mind-body medicine.

ENERGY IS THE CURRENCY OF LIFE

Worldwide, researchers now consider the body to be a hologram. What affects one part affects the whole holographic system. Furthermore, medical researchers refer to foods as biological response modifiers, because they either support or destroy cellular functions and energy production. The foods I recommend positively modify fatigue, exhaustion, mood and memory loss, but refined, processed and degraded foods give the natural terrain of your brain and body a terrible biological jolt—they are destructive biological response modifiers. They accelerate cellular confusion, cellular decline, cellular exhaustion and ultimately cellular blackouts earlier in your lifetime than you may be ready for. Tiredness is natural, but drop-dead fatigue is not.

FOUR EXAMPLES OF FOOD AS MEDICINE

Healthy food will always be the *present and future* of dynamic health and healing.If you are a peak performer, you need the best that food has to offer.

Let me present four examples: (1) how the simple flax seed and sesame seed are natural, powerful medicine; (2) how *greens+* startled veteran clinical researchers at the University of Toronto with remarkable success as food as medicine; (3) how fish oils boost your brainpower while reducing inflammation and depression; and (4) how green tea prevents cancer.

Example One: Flax Seeds and Sesame Seeds

Flax Lignans: Potent Anticancer Compounds

In addition to their high level of omega-3 fatty acids, flax seeds are also one of the most abundant sources of lignans. One study shows flax seeds contain seventy-five to eight hundred times the levels of the special lignan SDG than do other plant foods. The SDG lignan has proven to be the most bioavailable and effective of all lignans. Lignans are special compounds that are demonstrating some rather impressive health benefits, including positive effects in relieving menopausal hot flashes, as well as anticancer, antibacterial, antifungal and antiviral activity.

The most significant of these actions of lignans are their anti-cancer effects.

> Plant lignans are changed by the gut flora into *interolactone* and *enterodiol*, two compounds believed to be protective against cancer, particularly breast and prostate cancer.

Lignans are capable of binding to estrogen receptors and interfering with the cancer-promoting effects of estrogen on breast tissue. In addition, lignans increase the production of special sex hormone-binding compounds that regulate estrogen levels by escorting excess estrogen from the body via eliminative pathways.

Lignans Balance Estrogen Levels

Lignans are thought to be one of the protective factors against breast cancer in vegetarian women. Typically, women who excrete higher amounts of lignans in their urine (a sign of increased consumption) have much lower rates for breast cancer. High-lignan flax seeds may be the best choice for women going through menopause or for women at risk for breast cancer. It is currently estimated that as many as one in nine North American women will develop breast cancer. It is far superior to use flax seeds as medicine because they contain 100 mg of lignans per tablespoon. Flax seed oil may contain none, and if lignans are added back to flax seed oil—called high-lignan flax seed oil—it may only contain 10–25 mg per tablespoon of lignans. Lignans help by reducing the dangerous estrogens in the diet, balancing overall estrogen levels and thus reducing the risk of breast cancer.

> The researchers believe that the benefits are a result of the anti-estrogen effects of the lignans found in flax seed.

Flax Lignans Slow Breast Cancer Growth; Sesame Lignans Improve Immune Function

For women who already have breast cancer, flax seed can slow its progression. Researchers at the University of Toronto, Princess Margaret Hospital studied a group of thirty-nine women with newly diagnosed breast cancer tumors. The women received a muffin each day that contained 25 grams of ground flax seed, or a muffin that contained no flax seed. The researchers found that women who received the flax seed muffins experienced slower tumor growth and progression and a reduced risk of developing repeat breast cancer. Researchers feel that one of the reasons lignans may be so beneficial for fighting breast cancer is because the lignan structure is very similar to anticancer compounds such as Tamoxifen, which have antiestrogenic properties. Lignans are able to block excess estrogen.

Sesame Lignans—Powerful Medicine

Researchers are intrigued to discover that the three main lignans in sesame seeds—sesamol, sesamin and sesamolin—can favorably alter genes that cause your body to degenerate with age. Japanese researchers recently concluded that sesame lignans elevate both the alpha and gamma tocopherol fractions of vitamin E in the bloodstream by inhibiting an enzyme involved in breaking down vitamin E.

Amazingly, sesame lignans significantly reduce the risk factor for cardiovascular disease and high cholesterol by reducing the enzyme responsible for cholesterol biosynthesis. Furthermore, these lignans have antihypertensive effects and lower the risk of both heart attacks and strokes. Sesame lignans have a synergistic effect, enhancing the benefits of green tea EGCG, conjugated linoleic acid (CLA), and fish oils in promoting optimal fat burning and healthy weight. Finally, these lignans suppress system-wide inflammation, reduce the "bad" LDL cholesterol and prevent free radical lipid peroxidation of all good fats in your body, such as DHA and EPA from fish oil supplements.

Protect Yourself at Breakfast

I want you to follow my breakfast recommendation and grind 2 tablespoons of both organic flax seed and sesame seed, 30 grams of each, in a coffee grinder and add them to your breakfast protein shake. It is preferable to use freshly ground flax seed and sesame seed rather than packages of pre-ground seeds because once the packages are opened the ground seeds begin to degrade.

Example Two: *greens+*

greens+ is the result of 100 percent research and independent, double-blind clinical studies that have proven that it is a body-ready, cell-friendly food with exceptionally powerful abilities to defend your vitality and well-being.

- **Research #1:** Newly published research by Dr. Heather Boon, PhD, Pharmacist at the University of Toronto, has proven that *greens+* increases energy, vitality, mental health, well-being and overall health. These results were published in the prestigious *Canadian Journal of Dietetic Practice and Research* in August 2004.
- **Research #2:** A separate group of scientists at the University of Toronto demonstrated the potent antioxidant and cell-protection properties of *greens+*, documented in both test tubes and in a human clinical study published in the *Journal of Medicinal Foods* (2005). Medical researchers stated that, "Both *fat- and water-soluble* antioxidants were absorbed at an accelerated speed since the phosphatide complex in *greens+* has a hydrophilic, water-soluble fraction and a lipophilic, fat-soluble fraction." Dr. Venket Rao stated: "Overall, the results suggest an important role of *greens+* in reducing oxidative stress and prevention of chronic diseases."

  On April 7, 2003, the National Academy of Sciences board announced new recommended daily intake of choline, a supercritical B vitamin that is necessary to make your important brain messenger, acetylcholine. They suggest 425 mg of choline daily for adult women and 550 mg for adult men. Each serving of *greens+* supplies more than 466 mg of food-sourced, natural, bioavailable choline from the phosphatide complex, which is 26 percent phosphatidyl choline.
- **Research #3:** Dr. Najla Guthrie, PhD, demonstrated that "*greens+* achieved a *90 percent* reduction of lung cancer growth, and it was the only one of the three green foods examined to achieve a reduction in colon and lung cancer growth." This is powerful, essential and proven cell-friendly food as medicine.

- **Research #4:** A test called the Potential Renal Acid Load (PRAL) analysis determines a food's acid/alkaline effect inside the body. Your 100 trillion cells produce energy galore when they are alkaline, but energy blackouts when they are acidic. Researchers tested *greens+* against the most alkalinizing vegetable, spinach, and the most alkalinizing fruit, raisins, and discovered that *greens+* is 300 percent more alkalinizing than raisins and 200 percent more than spinach.
- **Research #5:** In yet another study, this one done at the Calcium Research Laboratory, associated with the University of Toronto Medical School and located at St. Michael's Hospital, Dr. Leticia Rao, PhD, the director of the lab, proved emphatically that "*greens+* can promote bone formation and protect against osteoporosis." These results were presented at the 31st annual meeting of the American Society of Bone and Mineral Research, in Seattle, to the best bone researchers in the world. Dr. Rao proved in her paper "Polyphenols in *greens+*™ and Bone Health" that the polyphenols—abundant micronutrients in natural food—can strengthen your bones and prevent bone loss. *The American Journal of Clinical Nutrition* wrote a comprehensive review about polyphenols preventing diseases associated with oxidative stress, including cancer, cardiovascular disease and neurogenerative disease.

Polyphenols are powerful micronutrients that you will be reading more and more impressive research about.

For more on these remarkable results, go to www.genuinehealth.com.

Example Three: Wild, Triple Fish Oils

Who would have believed it is possible that a unique fat in fish could have profound effects on your brain. Failure to eat enough of these special fats—called the long-chain omega-3 essential fatty acids EPA and DHA—are medically linked to an array of modern brainpower downturns: poor memory, low intelligence, attention-deficit disorder, poor vision, irritability, depression, dyslexia, inattention and learning disabilities.

How Fish Oil Creates Smarter Brains—Nutritional Neuroscience

Unquestionably, the brain is our most precious physical possession. Yet, the brain has received phenomenally little nutritional attention or intervention until now. Your brain cannot achieve top cognitive potential without adequate supplies of EPA and DHA omega-3 fatty acids from fish oils. An abundance of fish oil EPA and DHA fatty acids in the brain—at any age—can rejuvenate brain cells to construct the best neuronal architecture and biochemical wiring throughout your entire lifetime.

Your brain is 60 percent fat. EPA and DHA are long-chain dietary fatty acids, the most abundant omega-3 fatty acids in the brain and the most important fatty acids in the brain.

"Brain Smart" DHA

One fraction of fish oil, DHA, has been shown to enhance brainpower, memory, intelligence and attention span. Purdue University researchers have shown that DHA optimizes concentration, creativity and enthusiasm, as well as feelings of well-being. DHA is necessary for the prevention and management of attention-deficit disorder (ADD), attention-deficit hyperactivity disorder (ADHD) and learning disabilities, which, when corrected, lead to better brain function. DHA builds better brainpower, intelligence and a sharp memory. *The American Journal of Lipids* cited research that had a 60 percent success rate with ADHD using EPA- and DHA-rich fish oils. *The American Journal of Pediatrics*, in May of 2005, published the results of a large British study from Oxford University that got remarkable results in 40 percent of ADHD adolescents using fish oil supplements.

DHA can prevent, treat and reverse early-stage Alzheimer's disease, dementia, memory loss and learning disabilities, and increase intelligence, attention span, creativity and enthusiasm.

"Mood Smart" EPA

The other fraction of fish oil, EPA, is critical for maintaining superior mood stability and has therapeutic value in the prevention and management of inflammation, depression and mood swings. EPA tells your brain to feel good and is a mood elevator. Feel stressed out, anxious, moody or depressed? Try fish oils rich in EPA. The outcome of treating depression and irritability with the EPA fraction of fish oils far exceeded researchers' expectations. In both depression and postpartum depression, the brain cells need more omega-3 EPA to produce sufficient mood-regulating, messenger chemicals, according to Dr. Joseph R. Hibbelin, a research psychiatrist and fish oil authority at the National Institutes of Health in Bethesda, Maryland.

A Guide to Mighty Neuro-Supportive Brain Fats

The most important thing to remember is that your brain is growing, shaping and reshaping, changing every minute. It thrives on stimulation, exercise, learning, novelty and doing new things; such mental gymnastics actually encourage growth of new brain cell connections, enlarging memory, intelligence, good moods and learning capacity. In order to keep reshaping and growing favorably throughout your lifetime, and to prevent progressive mental decline, your brain requires fresh supplies of EPA and DHA fish oils daily.

Dr. Hibbelin says that cell membranes in the brain need to be pliable and fluid to perform the miracle of diverse communication. This is particularly true in the DHA-dependent synaptic gaps, the chemical bridges where nerve cells almost meet, but don't, and cell signals jump from one cell to another at speeds ranging from 1 to 150 miles per hour.

Every brain cell and its extensions, called dendrites, are covered by a delicate membrane that controls the cell's high-fidelity communication receptors, embedded deep in the membrane. The membrane's communication capability depends on the fluid consistency of this membrane. Only the DHA fraction of the fish oil gives brain cell membranes their soft, pliable texture to maximize your brainpower. Interestingly, the EPA fraction helps to reduce inflammation and help the membranes absorb DHA.

The best sources of ultra-pure, cold-water fish oils rich in EPA and DHA are the triple wild fish sources—anchovies, sardines and mackerel. These are small, clean fish from the pristine cold waters off the southern coast of South America. Another source is krill (*Euphausia superba*), a very small, Antarctic, shrimp-like zooplankton. Both sources are free of toxic metals, PCBs and dioxins. Unfortunately, the magazine *Nature* published research in the November 4, 2004, edition stating that both the density and distribution of krill in the Antarctic has declined by 70 percent since the 1970s because of declining winter ice, less chlorophyll to feed the krill and now excessive commercial fishing. Whale populations depend on krill for food, and there is not enough krill. I therefore do not recommend that you use krill oil.

It is important to note that fish oils are either steam or molecularly distilled to effectively remove any pollutants the fish may have accumulated. Fish oils are much safer and cleaner than eating fresh fish itself. If you are a vegan or strict vegetarian, use DHA called Neuromins™, extracted from micro algae.

North Americans are currently consuming only 130 mg of combined EPA and DHA daily—at least 520 mg short of the minimum 650 mg recommended by essential fatty acid experts like psychiatrists Dr. Hibbelin and Dr. Vincent DeMarco. The brain of an adolescent between the ages of eleven and seventeen needs a great deal more nurturing when it opens to higher functions and goes through a profound and rapid state of growth and change. This is a unique time to supplement with plentiful "mood smart" EPA and "brain smart" DHA essential fats to substantially increase good moods, attention span, brainpower and emotional stability.

PREVENT HEART ATTACKS AND CANCER WITH FISH OILS

"There is overwhelming evidence that EPA and DHA fish oils are clearly cardioprotective and are highly protective in preventing sudden cardiac death, death from heart disease and prevent certain arrhythmias. Epidemiological studies show a strong relationship between fish oil intake and reduced stroke risk because less carotid plaque is formed along arterial walls of daily fish oil users."

Circulation

> "Several test tube (in vitro) and animal studies have clearly shown that EPA and DHA from fish oil help to inhibit the promotion and progression of hormone-dependent cancers such as breast and prostate cancer."
>
> *American Journal of Clinical Nutrition*

Prenatal Nutrition

A woman's diet and lifestyle while pregnant, called fetal programming, can have a profound effect on the future mental and physical well-being of her child. Researchers have discovered that a mother's diet can even alter her child's gene functions without changing the DNA sequence, which plays a large role in the child's susceptibility to depression, ADD, ADHD, diabetes and cancer.

The Rowett Research Institute in Aberdeen, Scotland states that most of the EPA and DHA essential fats deposited in the growing fetus occur in the last ten weeks, or third trimester, of pregnancy. Furthermore, Dr. Bruce Holub and associates at the University of Guelph state, "Nutritional education of pregnant women's needs, to ensure adequate intake of fish oil EPA and DHA fats for optimal health of mother and child, and the inclusion of EPA and DHA in prenatal vitamins may be pertinent."

I am convinced that the single most important dietary influence for prenatal nutrition is adequate EPA and DHA omega-3 fats from enteric-coated triple fish oils. Make sure the softgels are specially protected with enteric-coating so they do not dissolve in the stomach but in your small intestine.

A Daily Brain-Boosting Formula

There is compelling scientific evidence that encourages us to take three fish oil capsules a day, one at each meal. On days when you are eating fresh salmon, mackerel or either sardines canned in olive oil or anchovies canned in their own oil, you do not need to take supplements.

To ensure you are receiving pure, clean EPA and DHA, I recommend you use a supplemental enteric-coated softgel from oils of wild mackerel, sardines and anchovies—the three most EPA- and DHA-rich fish oils.

Why Is Silent Inflammation So Dangerous?

Cholesterol reduction remained the Holy Grail of heart disease medicine until 2000, when elevated, silent inflammation levels, just below the perception of pain, were discovered to be the strongest, problematic component of heart disease, depression, cancer, arthritis, chronic pain, multiple sclerosis, dementia, Alzheimer's, ADD, ADHD and PMS.

The single most important thing you can do to keep silent inflammation under control is this: daily supplement with ultra-pure, high-dose omega-3 fish oils. Fish oils rich in EPA and DHA account for less than five percent of all supplement sales—and yet they are, along with "green drinks" the most important. Unlike vitamins and minerals, which last only a few hours in the bloodstream, EPA and DHA long-chain fatty acids from fish oils last several days. So you can take your daily dose all at once if that's easier.

EPA and DHA lower levels of silent inflammation, many years before, if not decades before, in advance of any serious health trouble. As an example, Ritalin only treats the symptoms of ADD and ADHD, but omega-3 fish oils treat the underlying cause—silent inflammation. You can test your inflammation status with your physician using the *Silent Inflammation Profile* (SIP) test that measures the ratio of arachidonic acid (AA) to EPA in the plasma phospholipids. Nutrasource Diagnostics, associated with the University of Guelph in Ontario is the testing laboratory and can be reached at (866) 637-8378 in Canada and (800) 404-8171 in the U.S. A good SIP result level is 3.0 and an ideal level is 1.5. Furthermore, reducing sugar consumption lowers excess insulin levels which lowers arachidonic acid (AA) formation, lowering your SIP.

Dr. Charlie Serhan of Harvard Medical School recently proved aspirin lowers inflammation by a process called aspirin-triggered epi-lipoxins with the strongest lipoxin being *resolvins*—the exact anti-inflammatory omega-3 fish oils make abundantly in your body. The most common blood tests for inflammation are high-sensitivity C-reactive protein (hs-CRP), homocysteine, fibrinogen and serum amyloid A (SAA), as well as the pro-inflammatory enzymes cyclo-oxygenase 2 (COX-2) and lipo-oxygenase (LOX)—all lowered with anti-inflammatory fish oils and by reducing insulin levels.

Important: Be sure to only use pharmaceutical grade, ultra-pure fish oil concentrates tested by the International Fish Oil Standards (IFOS) program administered by the University of Guelph. Find fish oils that are listed on the IFOS website at www.ifosprogram.com before purchasing any fish oil products, regardless of the advertising claims, since they must meet incredibly rigid IFOS standards for potency, label claim and purity. Two brands that receive the highest five star rating on the IFOS website are Genuine Health's (ehn inc.) entire line of condition-specific, ultra-pure omega-3 fish oils and Zone Labs Inc. Do not rely on short-chain essential fatty acids from flax seed oil which require nine very difficult biological steps to convert to the long-chain omega-3 essential fatty acids "mood smart" EPA and "brain smart" DHA that your body and brain need daily. Leap frog beyond these oils and use fish oils that are already long-chain, body-ready , inflammation lowering, essential fatty acids. Knowledge is power—when it comes to a lifetime of superior health.

Example Four: Green Tea

A landmark study published in the journal *Cancer Research* revealed mechanisms by which polyphenols, derived from green tea, not only help prevent the growth of tumors, but aid in preventing their spread. Green tea and black tea are derived from the same plant, *Camellia sinensis*. However, only green tea or Matcha green tea is rich in the flavonol group of polyphenols. The fermentation process used in making black tea destroys the biologically active polyphenols of the fresh leaf.

Of the four polyphenols, collectively called catechins, found in green tea leaves, epigallocatechin gallate (EGCG) has the strongest pharmacological activity to prevent prostate and breast cancer, and prevent the progression of all cancers by inhibiting metastasis, according to the British medical journal the *Lancet*. The antioxidant activity of green tea EGCG is about twenty-five to one hundred times more potent than vitamins C and E. One cup of green tea may provide 10 to 40 mg of polyphenols and has antioxidant activity greater than a serving of broccoli, spinach, carrots or the mighty blueberry.

Green Tea EGCG and CLA Promote Dramatic Weight Loss and Are Potent Cancer Protectors

A brand new study in the *American Journal of Clinical Nutrition* shows that green tea EGCG catechins reduce body fat in humans and use this fat to improve endurance. In twelve weeks of daily consumption of green tea polyphenols, abdominal fat was reduced 27 square cm versus 6 square cm in controls, as measured by computed tomography (CT) scans. Even better results are achieved when CLA is combined with green tea EGCG polyphenols.

University of Toronto Medical School researchers have shown that green tea EGCG polyphenols reduce body fat by 12 percent. CLA reduces body fat by 5 percent. Amazingly, the synergies of green tea polyphenols and CLA together do not combine as 12 + 5 = 17 percent body fat loss, but, astonishingly, as a *58 percent reduction* in body fat by reducing the proinflammatory PGE2 (prostaglandin E2) and elevating PGE1 and PGE3 to increase insulin sensitivity, reduce inflammation and promote fast fat burning. If you want to lose abdominal weight, try two capsules of *abs+* at each of your three meals. This will give you a total of 270 mg of EGCG green tea catechins and 3,400 mg of CLA. This is the exact amount and proportion of EGCG and CLA in the research. If, at each meal, you take one fish oil softgel that contains the "mood smart" EPA and the "brain smart" DHA, along with the preformed omega-6 fat from borage oil, the weight loss is accelerated even more. Dr. Henry Thompson at the AMC Cancer Research Center has shown CLA to be a potent inhibitor of morphological markers related to breast cancer. Dr. Ip and colleagues at the Roswell Park Memorial Cancer Center found that CLA is both anticarcinogenic and antimutogenic.

Part II

RESTORE

8

TEST-DRIVE THE SEVEN-DAY REJUVENATION PLAN

TAKE A TEST-DRIVE

I am eager for you to experience the thrill of having more zest, greater vitality, better mental clarity and improved brainpower. You will blast the blahs out of your life!

The promise of a notable difference in your robust vitality and overall mental performance in just twenty-one days may seem too good to be true. But if you eat exactly what I recommend for just twenty-one days, you will experience and see dramatic improvements and changes in how you feel and look, and positively respond to creative work or leisure.

This is a simple seven-day test-drive that will give you the joy of witnessing your very own transformation the healthy way.

If you follow my recommendations for a full twenty-one days, you will look younger, feel healthier and more vibrant, and be more mentally alert. Your special glow will return. Before you commit to a full twenty-one-day-long program, try the simple seven-day rejuvenation plan outlined in this chapter.

REMEMBER THIS IRREFUTABLE FACT

Eat only cell-friendly foods that will love you back.

This safe plan that I want you to follow is the same dietary strategy I use daily. I have successfully taught thousands of people—physicians, social workers, adolescents, parents, seniors, my family, my parents, health care professionals, gold-medal-winning Olympic athletes, teens rehabilitating from drug abuse, and internationally well-known entertainers—how to incorporate several simple approaches that give dazzling results beyond their expectations.

I worked with Randy Bachman, the lead guitarist from The Guess Who and Bachman Turner Overdrive (BTO), and when he animatedly and excitedly exclaimed to me, "I couldn't have imagined the remarkable difference seven days could make," I knew he had followed my suggestions. Randy's energy level, good mood and demeanor have been enthusiastically upbeat. He liked the robustly energetic, cheerful person he renewed in himself. He was and still is glowing with his youthful self-esteem intact. Randy lost 158 pounds in fourteen months, and his daughter lost 159 pounds without dangerous dieting. Now he knows how life was meant to be.

Old Ways
- declining stamina and energy
- midlife fatigue
- anticipated mental decline
- puffy skin and dull hair
- blues and blahs

New Ways
- endless, reassuring energy
- ageless, robust vitality
- boosting brainpower
- a youthful glow
- good moods all day long

YOU ARE ONLY AS GOOD AS YOUR LAST MEAL

The transformation on the road to remarkable energy and superior mental performance is just a single meal away. Master this book for beauty, robust vitality and a good brain.

YOUR SEVEN-DAY TEST-DRIVE BOOSTS CRAVE-BUSTING LEPTIN

The fat cells in your body manufacture an anti-craving, appetite-control hormone called leptin. If you secrete enough leptin into your bloodstream, it will quickly switch off your appetite so that you won't crave or binge on unhealthy foods.

Your brain cells use leptin in their communication network to regulate the degree of your appetite and the speed at which your body burns calories. Elevated leptin levels keep your calorie-burning metabolism running smoothly.

Leptin comes from the Greek derivative *leptos,* which means "thin." Your fat cells, as a survival mechanism, monitor the amount of food you eat. When fat cells determine that you have enough nourishment to sustain your well-being, they release leptin into the bloodstream and the brain quickly picks it up at the site of satiation and communicates powerful stop-eating orders. Leptin triggers production of a neuropeptide—alpha MSH—in the hypothalamus, the small area in the base of the brain that controls hunger and metabolism and sends a powerful metabolism booster signal to the brain to burn calories rather than store them.

TURN OFF YOUR APPETITE BETWEEN MEALS

leptin levels up = your appetite levels down =
no craving or bingeing

Break Craving and Bingeing Cycles with Leptin

Dr. Robert Atkins and I worked together on several occasions. I disagreed with his long-term approach to weight management, so we had lively scientific debates. I do not accept the low-carb approach. The healthiest strategy is a diet consisting of water, necessary healthy fats, lean protein and lots of low-density carbs (that is, carbs that are low on the glycemic index) from colorful vegetables, salad and moderate ripe fruit. Eating should leave you feeling nurtured, satiated and content.

I brought three critical points to Dr. Atkins's attention and explained why I thought he should adjust his approach. You can use these three points to your full advantage.

Point 1: If you cut out excessive fats, especially saturated fats from your diet, and eat a moderately low-fat diet, your leptin levels will stay elevated. Research cited in the *Diabetes Care* medical journal, the *Journal of Lipid Research*, the *American Journal of Clinical Nutrition* and the *International Journal of Obesity Related Metabolic Disorders* all present hard scientific evidence that a natural, lower-fat diet keeps appetite-busting leptin levels elevated, keeps you feeling full and prevents you from overeating.

Point 2: If you go on any typical low-calorie diet, your body misinterprets the diet as starvation, so your fat cells quickly slow down their leptin production, thus increasing your appetite. Within 72 hours of beginning any low-calorie diet, leptin levels drop by 50 percent of their previous level.

Rosemary described herself as a foodaholic. She had been dieting for one month when she suddenly found herself craving and bingeing, something she never did before. I asked Rosemary her ideal weight. She answered, "130 pounds." Multiply your ideal weight by twelve and the resulting number is the number of calories you need a day to boost leptin. Rosemary needs 130 × 12 = 1,560 calories as a minimum. If she goes below this, she cuts her leptin production.

Point 3: In a Harvard University study of 268 health professionals, men who exercised regularly had dramatically increased leptin sensitivity. This means that exercise makes your leptin levels work that much more effectively.

Suppress Your Excessive Appetite

Leptin plays a powerful role in appetite control, which research at Harvard, led by Dr. Barbara Kahn, further suggests may be due to its effects on the enzyme AMP-activated protein kinase (AMPK). Researchers describe AMPK as a "fuel gauge" that monitors cellular energy status.

A study published in the journal *Science* shows that leptin actually causes the brain to rewire itself. This research proved that leptin strengthened neural pathways that inhibited eating and weakened pathways that increased appetite.

THE SEVEN-DAY REJUVENATION PLAN

Wake Up

- Drink one to two 8-ounce glasses of water with a squeeze of fresh lemon, and drink it through a straw to reduce bloating from gulping too much air.

Fifteen Minutes Later

- Begin the day with a power shift, and put your body in an anabolic alkaline balance—this is the base to boost energy and brainpower all day long. Mix 1 tablespoon of a clinically proven *greens+ extra energy* or *Life Extension Herbal Mix* in either 8 ounces of water or in 6 ounces of water and 2 ounces of unsweetened pink grapefruit, orange, or black cherry juice. Mix in a plastic, hand-held tumbler and shake for 5 seconds. Sip and enjoy. If you do no other recommendation but this one, you will brighten your day with dynamic energy and stamina. It is today's version of your ancestors' wild greens and will prevent sluggishness all day long.

START EVERY DAY WITH A HEALTHY BREAKFAST

Let us get one thing established right from the beginning. A great day depends upon a great breakfast and high-octane fuel as healthy food all day long. Start your day with a dynamically balanced protein smoothie that I created for gold-medal-winning Olympic athletes.

THE ULTIMATE BREAKFAST POWER PROTEIN SHAKE

RECIPE

- 8 oz water, unsweetened rice milk, soy milk, hemp milk or organic, skim milk
- 2–4 heaping tablespoons of organic, low-fat plain soy or dairy yogurt
- 2 scoops of high-alpha whey protein isolate powder
- 1 full cup of any fresh or frozen berry, such as blueberries, blackberries or raspberries
- 2 tablespoons of both organic flax seeds and sesame seeds, 30 grams each, ground fresh in a coffee grinder for the lignan

fibers and the short-chain omega-3 fats

- ½ teaspoon of organic borage oil for the bioactive omega-6 fatty acid gamma linolenic acid, or simply swallow one 500 mg capsule of evening primrose oil for omega-6 fatty acids

Blend all ingredients in a blender for 10 seconds on low so that you do not denature the whey protein isolate powder.

- 1 softgel of enteric-coated concentrate wild, triple fish oil so that you get 300 percent better absorption and no fishy aftertaste. Use fish oils rich in EPA and DHA supercritical fats that your brain needs daily for good moods, enhanced memory and increased brainpower.

RECIPE NOTES

- Protein stimulates the release of the hormone glucagon, which maintains adequate levels of blood sugar (glucose) for the brain for optimal mental performance and acuity; it is the counter-regulatory hormone to insulin, so it will stabilize your blood sugar.

- The fish oils get dispersed in the preformed emulsions from the high-alpha whey protein isolate powder. These fat emulsions are an ideal delivery system to maximize fish oil absorption.

- Low-density carbohydrates that are low on the glycemic index, such as blueberries or any berry, give the low but steady glucose supply you require to maintain zest and robust energy by keeping insulin and neuropeptide levels in homeostasis—that is, in balance—throughout your body.

- Low-fat, unsweetened, plain organic yogurt supplies the friendly bacteria for your intestines.

MID-MORNING SNACK

- 1–2 cups of green tea, Matcha green tea or any herbal tea; stevia is the only allowable sweetener if you choose one
- a handful of celery, carrot and red pepper sticks

LUNCH

- 1 glass of water before meal (minimum, more if desired) with ½ tsp fresh lemon or lime juice
- lean plant-based or animal-based protein, such as:

- 3–4 oz of albacore tuna packed in spring water
- 4 oz of baked tempeh or firm tofu or 3 cups of beans or legumes such as edamame
- 3–4 oz of skinless, free-range chicken breast or thinly sliced turkey breast
- 4–5 oz of fat-free, dry curd cottage cheese
- 3 free-range poached eggs or a dry omelette (that is, made without oil in a non-stick pan) of 3 egg whites and 1 yolk (purchase only eggs of chickens that are fed a vegetarian diet that includes flax seeds)

- 3–4 cups of a colorful, zesty salad dressed with 2 tablespoons of extra virgin olive oil, a dash of fresh lemon juice to taste, a liberal sprinkle of a salt-free herbal seasoning, plus 2 drops of oil of oregano and 2 drops of oil of rosemary
- 1 triple fish oil, enteric-coated softgel from wild sardines, anchovies and mackerel
- 1 baked yam or sweet potato, topped with salsa

MID-AFTERNOON SNACK

- 2 cups of green tea, Matcha green tea, black tea or herbal tea; stevia is the only allowable sweetener if you choose one
- 1 serving of organic, colorful fruit such as an apple, prunes, peaches, oranges, black cherries, berries, melons, or pink grapefruit

DINNER

- 1 glass of water before meal (minimum, more if desired)
- 3–4 oz of steamed or grilled wild Northern B.C., wild Atlantic

or wild Alaskan salmon topped with fresh tarragon, watercress and diced sweet onion

- strict vegetarians can use unsalted tempeh, natto or firm tofu, whichever was not eaten at lunch
- 3 cups of 2 various colorful fresh vegetables steamed until they are crunchy tender, and drizzled with extra virgin olive oil
- sliced tomatoes, sliced cucumber, and sunflower sprouts dressed with 1 oz of dry-roasted pine nuts, sunflower seeds or pumpkin seeds
- a baked sweet potato or yam, baked squash or 1 cup of brown rice topped with unsweetened salsa

ALLOWABLE FOOD CHOICES

UNSWEETENED BEVERAGES

- clean water (8 glasses a day)
- green tea, Matcha or black tea (2 to 4 cups)
- rooibos (red leaves) or oolong tea
- herbal tea
- organic, skim milk
- rice, soy or hemp milk

PROTEIN SOURCES

- free-range eggs from chickens that are fed flax seed (high in DHA)
- wild salmon
- low-sodium, white, solid, water-packed albacore tuna
- sardines packed in olive oil
- unsalted whole seeds and nuts
- skinless chicken or turkey breast
- tempeh or natto
- extra-firm tofu (more protein, fewer carbs)
- fat-free, dry curd cottage cheese
- unflavored whey isolate or soy isolate protein powders or hemp protein, or plain enzymatically made rice protein powder

VERY LOW-DENSITY SALAD CARBOHYDRATES

- arugula
- Bibb lettuce
- mesclun lettuces
- watercress
- parsley
- curly endive
- dandelions
- escarole
- red or green leaf lettuce
- sunflower sprouts or broccoli sprouts
- green onions

LOW-DENSITY VEGETABLE CARBOHYDRATES

- asparagus
- broccoli
- kale
- Swiss chard
- red peppers
- beets and beet tops
- carrots

MEDIUM-DENSITY FRUIT CARBOHYDRATES

- blueberries
- blackberries
- raspberries
- strawberries
- black cherries
- stewed prunes
- apples
- melons
- peaches
- apricots
- plums
- pineapple
- mangoes
- papaya

NECESSARY FATS

- enteric-coated wild fish oil softgels, which are high in DHA and EPA from sardines, anchovies and mackerel, for long-chain omega-3 fats
- 6 macadamia nuts daily for omega-7 fats
- extra virgin olive oil for omega-9 fats
- borage oil or evening primrose oil capsules for biologically active omega-6 fatty acids

OTHER NECESSITIES

- fresh lemons
- salt-free herbal seasoning
- fresh herbs like oregano, basil, thyme and rosemary (garlic optional)
- oil of oregano
- oil of rosemary

THE SHOPPING LIST FOR THE TEST-DRIVE

Shopping for the foods in this list will give you a good opportunity to become familiar with your local natural food store. Please support these stores, which I call "health zones." Whenever possible, buy organic.

Here's what you need to prepare for your seven-day test-drive plan:

- seven 4 oz slices of fresh, wild salmon
- 1 container of *greens+ extra energy* **or** *Life Extension Herbal Mix*
- 1 dozen free-range eggs
- extra virgin olive oil
- 1 bottle of enteric-coated wild, triple fish oil softgels
- one 2 oz bottle of borage oil, or a small bottle of evening primrose oil capsules
- 7 cups fresh or frozen berries
- 7–14 servings of fresh colorful vegetables
- 7 servings of fresh fruit
- 32 fluid oz or 354 mL of unsweetened orange, red grapefruit

or black cherry juice
- colorful, fresh, crisp salad material emphasizing parsley, watercress and fresh herbs
- fat-free, dry curd cottage cheese
- tempeh or extra-firm tofu (if you choose the vegetarian option)
- salt-free herbal seasoning
- sardines in olive oil (if you choose this option at lunch)
- 4 skinless chicken breasts and 8 oz of thinly sliced turkey breast
- whey or soy isolate protein powder, or rice or hemp protein powder
- organic, skim milk
- rice, soy or hemp milk
- 1 container of low-fat plain organic yogurt

Now is the time to stand up and be counted. A good start would be to test-drive this seven-day plan in your daily lifestyle and dietary strategy with balance, variety and moderation. Whether you are a "tiptoer" or a "plunger," begin now.

The Seven-Day Rejuvenation Plan puts the proof right where it belongs—right in your hands. All you have to do is be consistent! Follow as faithfully as you can the following principles, which will boost your radiant vitality and brainpower.

The favorable outcome of the Seven-Day Rejuvenation Plan is based on your following these eight principles as best as you can. All you have to do is be consistent.

---

1. Eat three meals and two snacks a day. Do not eat after 8:00 p.m. or rising insulin levels will prevent deep sleep.
2. Balance your protein-to-carbohydrate ratios at each meal. Eat sufficient protein at each meal.
3. Eat natural, low-density carbohydrates, not processed, high-density carbohydrates.
   NOTE: You require 5 grams (1 teaspoon) of sugar (glucose) circulating in your bloodstream every 4 hours for robust good energy

(your liver keeps serum glucose levels at 0.1 percent). Only cell-friendly whole foods keep your bloodstream properly balanced with glucose.

4. Eat colorful, in-season, organic (when possible) fruits, vegetables, salads, sea vegetables, spices and herbs as your low-density carbohydrate energy source. Consume 40 grams of fiber daily.
5. Pre-hydrate with eight glasses of clean water throughout the day.
6. Have enteric-coated fish oil softgels, *plus* a GLA source such as evening primrose or borage oil, *plus* extra virgin olive oil, *plus* ground flax seeds, *plus* ground sesame seeds, *plus* six to ten macadamia nuts daily.
7. Avoid sugars, excess salt, fried foods, hydrogenated or semi-hydrogenated oils (trans-fatty acids), vegetable oils, food colorings, food additives and MSG.
8. Get 7 to 9 hours of sleep a night in a dark environment to allow for a good hormonal cascade to produce your deep-sleep hormone melatonin. Once melatonin is secreted, it lowers your body temperature by 1.5 degrees Fahrenheit. This cooling then allows human-growth hormone (hGH) to be produced by your pituitary gland in spurts during deep sleep all night long. Critical hGH is the hormone that revitalizes your 100 trillion cells so they renew, restore and regenerate. You can increase critical hGH by increasing deep sleep. By age fifty, most people's hGH has been reduced by a startling 40 percent because of severe sleep debt.

Salad Dressing on the Seven-Day Plan—Why?

The right foods act as anti-inflammatory, skin-glowing cosmetics for our facial skin, body skin and, surprisingly, shiny and lustrous hair. Food is much more than just a life-sustaining, life-giving, energizing substance. Food is our single most powerful antiaging tool. The many choices we make daily—or even hourly—immediately influence not only our vital energy and critical mental performance, but also our appearance.

The wrong oils and fats directly influence the growing number of wrinkles and amount of sagging in your face, as well as your drooping skin texture, enlarged pore size, dull skin tone, and under-eye bags and puffiness. You can reverse and certainly prevent visible skin damage and put your best face forward by using the oils and salad dressing I use and highly recommend.

Working from the inside out, by using the right oils, the right antioxidants and quality phytonutrients in natural foods—as well as quality supplements—will produce striking short-term and cumulative long-term improvements to refresh your skin cells.

I want you to incorporate cold-pressed, extra virgin olive oil into your diet and salad dressing on a daily basis. Olive oil is the type of fat that lowers harmful LDL cholesterol at the same time as it raises the level of heart-protective HDL cholesterol. Olive oil is the only safe, stable oil that does not require refrigeration.

Use cold-pressed, extra virgin olive oil daily. Your skin will glow and your energy will soar. The results are nothing short of miraculous. Olive oil offers an unmatched myriad of defenses.

My favorite organic, cold-pressed, extra virgin olive oil is Biolea, from a fifth-generation family's organic olive grove in Greece. Contact the family at rawthyme@yahoo.ca or (250) 748-7385.

Olive oil contains 75–82 percent of a non-essential monounsaturated fatty acid called oleic acid, a member of the omega-9 family. Oleic acid offers an entire spectrum of beneficial services. It:

- does not readily oxidize, is stable, and does not produce free radicals
- is transported into the cell plasma membrane, helping to maintain the structural integrity of neuronal membranes
- acts as a regulator in the cell plasma membrane to ensure that EPA- and DHA-rich omega-3 fish oil fats penetrate the cell membrane to keep the lipid bilayer subtle, fluid and stabilized
- helps intestinal absorption of nutrients
- supports gallbladder activity
- prevents water-retention edema
- reduces the risk of both breast and prostate cancer
- contains antioxidants, in particular the four most powerful polyphenols—tyrosol, hydroxytyrosol, verbascoside and

oleuropein—which are found only in cold-pressed, extra virgin olive oil and give olive oil its slightly bitter taste; hydroxytyrosol prevents the oxidation (the equivalent of rusting) of keratin protein, making your hair soft, shiny and radiant

Sam's Savory Salad Dressing

- 2 tablespoons per person of cold-pressed, extra virgin olive oil (organic, if possible)
- 1 teaspoon of fresh lemon or lime juice to taste or ¾ teaspoon of unfiltered, unpasteurized apple cider vinegar; alternate between these two
- several drops of both oil of oregano and oil of rosemary
- liberal sprinkle of a salt-free herbal mix seasoning and turmeric
- a dash of flaked or granulated Nova Scotia dulse
- 1 teaspoon of gomasio (dry-roasted organic sesame seeds)
- 1 clove of finely chopped garlic or a dash of non-irradiated garlic seasoning (garlic is an optional ingredient)
- ½ teaspoon of clean, pure water
- 1 tablespoon of miso

EAT MINDFULLY

Your mealtimes can be a downtime of comfort, nourishment and healing or quite the opposite—extremely detrimental. Unfortunately, many people today eat at the same breakneck speed they use for everything else. If you are depressed, anxious, angry or distracted when eating, your body will not digest or assimilate your food well, and you will not receive the revitalization you need. It is vitally important to switch on a rhythm of mindful calm while eating slowly and savoring your food, and switch off potentially upsetting things like the news, business discussions or major dilemmas. I am guilty of old eating habits as I tend to eat fast, but I have made an effort to change my eating habits.

I have found that if I say a grace or thanksgiving before my meals or snacks, I slow down my fast-paced rhythm. Grace or a thanksgiving remind us to be grateful and we can be more conscious of what we eat and how we eat it, using voluntary calorie restriction to keep our energy currency available all life long. This is a good part of your personal plan for becoming a Wise Elder.

9

FOUR TIPS TO ENERGIZE YOUR DAY—TODAY!

IMPROVE YOUR PERFORMANCE AND SHARPEN YOUR MIND

Today's Energy Crisis

Fatigue is no longer an inevitable consequence of living. Every day, as reported by Dr. Burrios-Chapin and colleagues in the journal *Stress Medical* in 1997, almost 70 percent of adults suffer an energy crisis, a drop-dead fatigue from trying to navigate a day full of must dos as they become victims of what Dr. Joey Shulman likes to call "the incredible shrinking day." Their minds keep telling them to keep going, but their bodies are screaming, "I can't, I'm exhausted."

Please don't let anyone convince you that fatigue is all in your head, or even worse, that you need antidepressants for it.

Are You Tired of Being Tired?

I have completed revolutionary energy research analyzing peak performers for years, and I'd like to reveal the secrets of their endless reserve of high-quality energy.

You can learn to beat fatigue and restore your energy in seven days with great results, and in twenty-one days with remarkable results.

It is easy to get all the energy you need. Impossible? It may have been in the past, but not now. A daily energy crisis—feeling weak and depleted, sputtering and stalling—is not natural and you don't have to be condemned to a life of chronic exhaustion.

You have home and bill responsibilities, children and/or aging parent responsibilities and career responsibilities. You have to drag yourself out of bed and all day long it feels like riding a bike uphill with two flat tires. You feel tired, draggy, even downright sleepy.

I was in the CBC radio station studios in Calgary, doing a live call-in radio talk show called Wild Rose. A lawyer from Montana phoned in and said, "Sam, I'm exhausted, and all the little things I enjoy—exercise classes, socializing, gardening, playing with my two sons—all came to a meltdown, a screeching halt. I had to give up everything I like to do to have the energy for what I have to do—going to work, preparing cases, going to court, paying bills—all the while trying to run a busy household." She continued, "I feel dead tired, I'm running on empty, always struggling with bleak depression. I feel terribly trapped by sickening exhaustion due to circumstances, pressing obligations, an unending load of family chores and parental duties that nobody but I can do."

CAN YOU RELATE TO ANY OF HER EXHAUSTION AND FATIGUE?

Let me be clear for her and for you. It does not have to be this way any longer. You can be energized and happy.

Here's what I told my caller.

A NATURAL ENERGY BOOST...BETTER ENERGY

Fast-Acting Energy Tip #1: Use food supplements to ignite all-day-long energy.

Your thyroid gland is the ultimate regulator for efficient energy production all day long.

The lobes of this small, butterfly-shaped gland at the base of your neck, just below the Adam's apple, fit on either side of your windpipe. The thyroid makes only *one teaspoon of hormones each year*, yet this tiny amount can absolutely make or break your energy levels.

Why? Because your energy levels are determined by the rate at which your body metabolizes food into energy and that rate is regulated by your thyroid. A sluggish thyroid means a sluggish metabolism and energy dysfunction at the cellular level, which results in poor digestion, constipation, lowered mood and depression, and decreased cognitive function. The only way to maintain a well-functioning thyroid is to have a sufficient amount of the free, unbound amino acid tyrosine in your system.

- Tyrosine is your main factor in making energy.
- Tyrosine supports good, balanced metabolism rates so you have a steady supply of energy.
- Tyrosine has an even greater impact on your energy metabolism by being converted to, and increasing, the hormone dopamine, your powerful hormone for maintaining robust, balanced energy all day long.
- Elevated tyrosine levels lower chronic fatigue states.
- Tyrosine eliminates brain exhaustion and fatigue.
- Tyrosine requires a combination of vitamin C and pyridoxine HCl (vitamin B6) to convert it to your ergogenic (dynamic) hormone dopamine, which quickly lifts your enthusiasm, creativity and production. Dopamine is your get-up-and-go hormone.

It turns out that many people over twenty-four years of age lack tyrosine in their diet because of poor-quality protein intake or because they can't absorb protein due to digestive problems.

Tyrosine is not a replacement or substitute for thyroid medication, but an ideal complement to it.

A Natural Solution for "Brain Fog"

By the age of thirty-four your cells begin to lose their full capacity to produce energy, and by around age thirty-eight to forty your brain cells start to become energy-starved, so your brain seems foggy.

A second amino acid, taurine, can be supplemented to ignite more and better "high-fidelity" brain cell communication network messengers in your brain's neurons.

As if that weren't good enough, taurine increases the exercise time to exhaustion and maximal workload in adults by lowering acid-causing lactic acid. It enables you to exercise longer and more efficiently. You become more alkaline. Taurine helps to retain the cardio-protective minerals potassium and magnesium. Therefore, it strengthens your heart, which is important because the heart pumps 13,000 pints of fluid throughout the body each day—over 60,000 miles of blood vessels. Taurine reduces your irritability, insomnia, migraines, cravings and depression. Furthermore, a third amino acid, glycine, helps to synthesize the brain's inhibitory, calming and soothing neurotransmitter GABA, which regulates excitatory nerve fibers and pathways in the brain, called glutamergic fibers, so you feel enthusiastic, alert and motivated, but not wired.

Herbs Boost Vitality

The herbs rhodiola rosea, kola nut, gotu kola, astragalus and suma are classic adaptogenic herbs that both reduce mental and physical fatigue and increase cognitive performance. They increase energy (ATP) production within the "energy factories," the tiny mitochondria of each of your 100 trillion cells. These powerful herbs increase the neuro-supportive effects of acetylcholine, the neurotransmitter messenger that ferries information quickly and efficiently from cell to cell within the brain. Amazingly, these herbs give you a natural mental, emotional and mood boost that can last for 5 to 6 hours.

Boosting Energy Naturally—A Better Alternative to Coffee

Your 100 trillion cells are concerned with only two goals: producing abundant energy, and surviving. So in order to help your cells do what they do best, you must feed them cell-energizing foods that give them the necessary energy to keep your organs at peak performance, your brain sharp, your memory impeccable, your heart pumping, your lungs working efficiently, your stomach digesting and absorbing food, your immune system vigilant and your mood boosted.

Your cells cannot choose between cell-energizing or cell-exhausting foods they receive—only you can. Wisely choose a cutting-edge supplement to boost your energy. Rejuvenating your body's vigorous energy system by deliberately bolstering it with nature's most reinvigorating amino acids, energy-supportive herbs (kola nut, gotu kola, suma, rhodiola rosea and astragalus) and power-packed foods will powerfully energize you today, tomorrow and all life long.

The kola nut (*Cola nitida*) is a seed kernel related to the cacao plant (the source of chocolate) and is native to the rain forests of West Africa and now cultivated in the West Indies. The nut contains up to 3 percent natural caffeine combined with plant fibers, vitamins, minerals and antioxidants. Research by Dr. R.R. Griffiths of Johns Hopkins University and Dr. H.R. Lieberman of the U.S. Army Research Institute supports that a modest dose of 100 to 200 mg of naturally derived caffeine daily can be energizing, enhance memory, increase alertness and boost your motivation, good mood and creative production.

The kola nut is a member of the cacao family of plants, and a rich source of the family of antioxidants called pentameric procyanidins (pentamer). Dr. Robert Dickson, professor of oncology at Georgetown University, explains that pentamer is a potent anticancer, antimutagenic compound that initiates apoptosis (death) to cancer cell colonies.

Don't Leave Home Without Them

- energy boost: 80 mg of naturally occurring caffeine from the kola nut plus the herbs rhodiola rosea, gotu kola, astragalus and suma and the mineral chromium that boost energy production
- energy extension: the amino acids taurine, glycine and tyrosine, the vitamins B6 and C, and the herb rhodiola rosea enhance stamina and concentration
- energy recovery: the amino acids taurine and glycine, vitamin C, and the herbs astragalus and rhodiola rosea balance your adrenal glands and prevent a mood downturn

Fast-Acting Energy Tip #2: Use "brain friendly" EPA and DHA fats for both brains and beauty.

Your brain uses only long-chain, not short-chain, omega-3 fatty acids.

Wisely leapfrog way ahead by using preformed, brain ready, biologically active, long-chain omega-3 fatty acids from fish oils. Flax oils are good, but are made only of short-chain omega-3 fats (however, while they add nothing to brain function, in moderation they are good for healthy skin and cardiovascular health). As mentioned earlier in Chapter 7, the best sources are wild, cold-water anchovy, mackerel and sardines, all small clean fish. Remember, always purchase fish oil softgels that are enteric-coated so they do not dissolve in your stomach, but in your small intestine so you have no fishy aftertaste.

Use fish oil capsules that deliver both EPA and DHA fats together and that are pharmaceutical grade and molecularly distilled. These fats also make your facial skin structure more radiant and wrinkle-free. They improve intelligence and brain function.

Research shows that to achieve a powerful "brain booster," the essential fatty acid EPA should be in a 1 to 2.5 ratio with DHA. Ideally you want 100 mg of EPA to 250 mg of DHA to create greater mental energy and enhanced overall cognitive performance. The EPA actually facilitates the absorption of DHA and improves cellular function.

Neurotransmitters and hormonal systems in the brain do not operate independently of one another. They cross-talk, or communicate with each other, at speeds of up to 150 miles per hour. To travel quickly, without delay or lapses, stable, pliable DHA fatty acids form at the ends of each neuron, and in the inside wall of each brain cell, called the lipid bilayer. DHA acts as an energy circuit for the brain, to allow it to operate at warp speed. EPA allows DHA to be absorbed into the lipid bilayer of neurons.

EPA alleviates depression and inflammation. DHA enhances pure brainpower.

Trying to maintain radiant vitality and brain function without adequate DHA and EPA is like trying to start your car with no oil or gas. Without adequate DHA and EPA, your brain, mood and memory cannot function properly and cannot form new neural connections, let alone repair and maintain old ones. Recent research indicates that only DHA, with the help of EPA, can stimulate the growth of new brain nerve cells. Dr. Michael A. Schmidt, in *Brain-Building Nutrition*, states "this explains why DHA is preferentially transported across the placenta into the fetal circulation for maximum support of brain development in the child."

How to Cause an Instant Surge in Your Brainpower

Dr. Alan C. Logan, ND, of New York City, author of the soon to be published book *The Brain Diet*, has published a number of articles on omega-3 fatty acids and mood that have received international attention. His most recent article, "Omega-3 Fatty Acids: A Primer for the Mental Health Professional," is the most requested article in the prestigious journal *Lipids in Health and Disease*. This article is now available at www.genuinehealth.com. While in the graduate neuroscience program at the University of Hartford, Dr. Logan published his hypothesis that omega-3 fatty acids may influence the production of a chemical called brain-derived neurotrophic factor (BDNF), which can help the brain develop new brain cells, even into adulthood. Dr. Logan formulated a dynamic, molecularly distilled fish oil capsule called *o3mega+ think*, which is the perfect ratio of 100 mg of EPA to 250 mg of DHA, for a remarkable energizing brain boost. Check it out at www.ifosprogram.com.

Fast-Acting Energy Tip #3: Oxygenate your 100 trillion cells.

Oxygenate your deep tissues and 100 trillion cells throughout the day. Your energy, mental clarity and euphoria increase dramatically when you recharge your cells with cell-friendly, refreshing oxygen and expel all the toxic carbon dioxide.

Twice a day, breathe slowly and deeply through both nostrils for one minute to turn on your parasympathetic nervous system to reduce emotional, mental and physical anxiety by 70 percent.

Most people use only one-third of their lung capacity, so their 100 trillion cells never get enough oxygen to create the proper combustion to produce energy galore. Chapter 13 covers deep, re-energizing breathing techniques that are simple to use.

THE BENEFITS OF DEEP BREATHING

- enhances energy
- stabilizes emotions
- improves moods
- boosts alertness
- makes skin more radiant
- revitalizes deep tissues
- improves brainpower
- reduces physical fatigue
- de-stresses anxiety
- reduces mental exhaustion

Remember

You can live: **thirty days** without food
four days without water
four minutes without oxygen

Open Wide

Feel a yawn coming on? Go for it. "Your brain is telling you that you need more oxygen," states Allen Elkin, PhD, author of *Stress Management for Dummies*. But learn to yawn correctly: "We're all too polite about it and don't get enough oxygen in." Inhale deeply through a wide-open mouth, taking the breath all the way down to your belly. Exhale fully through your mouth. Yawning properly is an energy booster and a bonus stress reducer.

Breathe Energy-Boosting Aromatherapy Scents

Certain scents, including peppermint, rose, coffee, cinnamon, chocolate and vanilla, can boost your energy and attention span. "Odor appears to hit areas of the brain that affect attentiveness, judgment and planning," writes Joel Warm, PhD, co-author of *Psychology of Perception*. A natural incense, even a natural essential oil-scented soap or bath, may brighten up your brain. My favorite revitalizing and detoxifying bath salt recipe is:

10 drops of grapefruit seed extract
10 drops of juniper

10 drops of laurel
6 drops of cypress
1 cup (250 mL) Dead Sea salts or Epsom salts

Fast-Acting Energy Tip #4: Keep your body, spine, neck and head in fluid balance and alignment.

An out-of-alignment body, vertebra, spine or neck can throw off your core balance and core energy. Can you drive safely and effectively if your steering wheel is totally bent out of shape or if your tires are moving in four different directions? Ninety-eight percent of all drivers responding to the Rand Institute Survey of Drivers rated themselves in the top 5 percent of drivers, when in fact not all of them could be, so please don't overestimate your wellness if your core balance is off. You may not be in the top 5 percent of peak-performing energizers.

I had just finished running 10 miles in 52 minutes when I first arrived on Salt Spring Island, British Columbia in the autumn of 1995. I ran across a large wet cedar deck, in heavy rain, and hydroplaned out of control into a railing, instantly breaking five ribs and falling over the railing head first. I landed 15 feet below, upside down, on my neck, on a rocky outcrop. I lost my speech, vision and hearing for three days. I shattered four vertebrae in my neck. Only because of the brilliant, cutting-edge care of Dr. Aslam Khan, DC, and the remarkable pain-control injections of prolotherapy by Dr. Nasif Yasin, was I able to fully recuperate. They are at Optima Health Solutions International in Vancouver, British Columbia, and their information is in the Medical Resource section of this book. You can find them at www.optimahealthsolutions.com.

These dedicated, revolutionary health care providers, like so many others across North America that are listed at the back of this book, are at ground zero in initiating integrative medicine as a standard protocol. Dr. Khan, as an example, worked on my cranio-sacral system, which involves the brain, neck, spinal cord and cerebrospinal fluid, and quickly relieved and balanced my neurological complications. He has developed an absolutely revolutionary device called the Khan Kinetic Therapy that changes your *primary energy mechanism* while you comfortably recline. His methodology is based on the principle that the body is structurally and functionally one reciprocally interrelated system.

The Mind-Body Energy Connection

Researchers at Boston's Forsyth Institute and at Harvard University have studied the human embryo to determine the mind-body energy connection. They have found that when an embryo consists of just four cells, an electric gradient starts switching on genes. A power switch is turned on that begins to animate you to life.

The study of embryological development shows that the brain is the very first organ to develop. The brain then sends energy through the spinal cord and nerves to create and energize all your trillions of cells and every organ in your body. From that point on, your brainpower flow continues to control all functions and healing in the body for the rest of your life. As a result, if there is any interference, mechanical restriction or damage to the spinal cord or the nervous system, there will be communication network malfunction and interruption in the robust vitality or healing energy to your organs, tissues and cells.

You Need to Be Plugged In

A healthy brain and spinal cord float in a liquid called the cerebrospinal fluid—what Dr. Khan calls "the ocean of life." My personal problems were specifically in the brain stem, the place where electrochemical impulses and signals are transferred between the brain and the body. The brain stem and spinal cord connect at the thalamus like a two-pronged plug at the end of an extension cord. These two prongs regulate both the sympathetic and parasympathetic nervous systems.

Improvements in the alignment and proper curvature of your neck and spine is evidence that you are not only feeling energized and well, you *are* well. Regular massages help to keep you aligned and relaxed, loosen deep tension and prevent acute stress from accumulating in muscle tissue, as well as remove both physical and emotional toxins.

Seek out a high-quality chiropractor, naturopathic doctor, osteopath, acupuncturist, podiatrist or physiotherapist if you have any misalignments. From my twenty-five years of professional experience, let me please say this: assume that you have several misalignments and do not hesitate to get back in alignment. Keeping your vital life force flowing freely as on-demand dynamic energy is a critical part of integrative medicine.

10

MY SECRETS TO A HAPPY LIFE

BE KIND

Think about your day today. Did you allow your mind-body energy centers to flow in a restricted manner or an unrestricted manner? When I have the opportunity to motivate people and see them happy and full of healthy self-esteem and social esteem, I know that I have done my job. When we lift our minds to that unrestricted universal energy, we create peace and happiness in the world. The most remarkable part about this universal energy is that because we have it in abundance, we cannot help but share it with others. The more we share it, the more we have; it causes a chain reaction of reciprocated kindness.

> "When one door of happiness closes, another opens; but often we look so long at the closed door that we do not see the one which has been opened for us."
>
> Helen Keller

HAVE A HAPPY HEART

We can all gain a happy heart and optimism by nurturing close relationships. "Simply looking at the picture of someone you love can dampen stress responses," states Alexandar Radan, MD. A recent study reported that thinking of supportive family or friends for a few minutes before a final exam helped participants minimize increases in heart rate and blood pressure.

Cardiologist Harvey Zarren, medical director of the Healing Your Heart program at Union Hospital in Lynn, Massachusetts, used to apply a variation of this technique when he rode in the ambulance with heart patients. He would ask the patient to discuss the thing or person he or she loved most. As if by magic, high blood pressure fell and abnormal heart rhythms diminished. His patients never had a cardiac arrest in the ambulance. Given that heart disease is still the nation's leading killer, we could all benefit from a happy heart.

Major lifestyle changes are not necessary for a happy heart response. Even little ones help. Ten minutes of meditation a day can prevent a heart attack in the long run, and in the short run can fill our hearts with gratitude and optimism. Consistency of practice is more important than duration. Next is exercise. Simply putting on a pair of sneakers and walking is an ideal way to refresh your heart and reduce sadness.

Jackson Brown, formerly of the Eagles, in one of his songs sings a line that says we've left it up to someone else to be the one to care. Some of us don't want to be the one to care, even about ourselves. We just want to run and hide from responsibilities to our family and the world because sometimes we feel overwhelmed. That is why I feel so compelled to say that happiness does not belong only to a chosen few—it belongs to you. It was given to you as your birthright. You only have to claim it, or maybe reclaim it.

TATTOOS, SHAMPOOS AND BARBECUES

Just as your perception of tattoos, shampoos and barbecues determine your opinion for or against each one, likewise your happiness is 100 percent based on your perception of yourself.

Do you know why you are unhappy? You may say it is due to loneliness, your job or your relationship. There is only one cause of unhappiness: the false beliefs we keep in our minds, beliefs so widespread in society that it never occurs to us to question them. You may not even suspect that your beliefs and programming are wrong and distorted. Don't blame yourself, blame your perceptions—and decide that it is time to change them. There is no reality, there are only perceptions of it.

The psychologist Abraham Maslow was a pioneer in studying the positive aspects of human personality and behavior. Maslow talks about the need to reconcile our life, and to grow, change and transform our perceptions to "peak experiences" that carry with them extraordinary curative power. One taste of this peak experience can make life undeniably understandable and beautiful. It is a life power in its purest form. It is not energy or strength or insight or genius, but the power that underlies all of these. People who dare to transform state that there is incredible order existing everywhere; there is no chaos in the mind or body or world.

The complexity of the mind-body connection is misleading. What emerges from this complexity are clear images and perceptions of reality, just as coherent as the television images that are made from thousands of individual dots. False perceptions of ourselves, or ourselves in the world, disintegrate when we analyze them. If not, false perceptions form a barrier no thick metal door could possibly match. Albert Einstein himself experienced this awareness. He testified to moments when "one feels free from one's own identification with human limitation." These transformations happen in a state of silence when you have no control over this awareness, but it is by no means only emptiness. Maslow and Einstein realized the universe in themselves. We all need to become Einsteins of a new consciousness and perception that the mind and body are not limited.

The first western scientist to make a major breakthrough like this was American physiologist Robert Keith Wallace. Within a few minutes of beginning to meditate, his subjects entered a state of deep relaxation in the 8 Hz range in their EEGs, marked by slower breathing and heartbeat, and decreased oxygen consumption in their breathing. Their bodies' metabolic rates had dropped into a metabolic reduction called a hypometabolic state. It takes 4–6 hours after falling asleep to reach this hypometabolic state, whereas meditators took only a few minutes and their metabolic rates were 100 percent lower. His subjects reported feelings of relaxation with alertness, inner silence, and peacefulness. Wallace was legitimizing the mind-body connection. Most amazingly, he realized that we can control the physical life process and mental perceptions that constantly influence us every minute, whether we realize it or not. Wallace's research showed him that what we believe, we are—and will become. It adds another dimension of unbounded reality in which we can make this world a heaven or a hell.

We all have the power to make a new reality, born of new, enlightened perceptions. We tend to forget that peace, contentment, compassion, love and fulfillment are the actual norm. Make the transformation yourself and enjoy this remarkable experience— it will give you enough power to last a lifetime.

FEEL GOOD

When you decide to put your heart into something, dynamic energy flows. Once you visualize yourself as empowered—once you truly believe in yourself and the inexhaustible Divine spark that burns unrelentingly in all of us alike—your mind, emotions and heart will have done their part. Get your body ready to be a lively electric grid and transfer this dynamic energy, happiness and creativity into the joy of being alive, and better serve the world.

> "There is no duty we so much underrate as the duty of being happy. By being happy, we sow anonymous benefits upon the world."
>
> Robert Louis Stevenson

I just took a break from writing to go out to my large organic vegetable garden that grows beautifully in raised beds. The late season sunflower heads and all the leaves were turned toward the sun, the Source of light and life. Do not turn away from your spiritual Source, believing you could exist without it.

There is a tremendous difference between information, understanding and wisdom. Today we've gained enormous understanding of our world through a bounty of information, but we've lost the wisdom of how we fit into the world.

We used to know better. We've flouted the rules and we feel unfulfilled because we have lost faith in our own innate wisdom—and it just might be time to get it back!

DAILY MEDITATION

Comfort, hope, optimism, fulfillment, joy, inner peace, a deep sense of well-being—sacred texts have long promised such rewards to the faithful. According to Dr. Harold Koenig, a co-director of the Center for Spirituality, Theology and Health at Duke University, from 2000 to 2002 more than one thousand scholarly articles on the relationship between religion and mental health were published in academic journals, as opposed to just one hundred from 1980 to 1982. Even if you compare two people who have symptoms of depression, the more spiritual person will be less sad. Studies show that the more people incorporate spirituality into daily living—attending services, reading Scripture, praying, meditating—the better off they appear to be on two measures of happiness: frequency of positive emotions and an overall sense of satisfaction with life. The sense of unshakable faith and the truth of one's beliefs are most closely linked with life contentment, fulfillment and satisfaction.

I meditate twice each day. It soothes my being and allows me to feel more connected to the human family and the world around me. It leaves me calm, but exuberant and alert. I walk around with a lighter step, feel enormous gratitude for life and feel a sense of collective blessedness. To my surprise, meditation actually allows me to be more productive in my work.

CONTRIBUTE TO GLOBAL WELLNESS

It is self-evident that the best society increases human happiness and reduces human misery. We in North America feel vaguely dissatisfied even though we have what we want, vaguely guilty for wanting more material success for ourselves and our children, and vaguely disappointed because it didn't fulfill as advertised.

To begin fresh anew, we must say goodbye to who we once were.

Today we live in a society in which there is no agreed-upon philosophical basis for public policy or private morality. Pragmatic policymakers claim to be doing "what works," but works to what end? We are past the period of evolution when only the fittest can survive. We are in the period of the survival of the wisest and we need to give less value to status and pursuit of personal pleasure, and more value to global wellness. We should rededicate ourselves and our society to the pursuit of love, compassion, kindness, hope, optimism and equality rather than the goal of dynamic efficiency. This idea is not new, but it is taking a real beating in the current era of unrestrained individualism.

We need to gaze at the big scoreboard and be inspired to think of global happiness, global ecology and global wellness. We need a radically new, worldwide view—beginning with ourselves.

A RADICALLY NEW WORLD VIEW

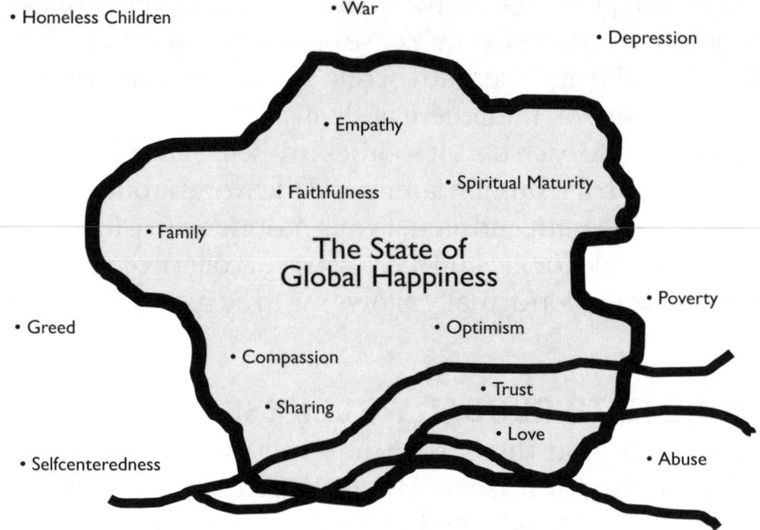

TAKE A CREATIVE QUANTUM LEAP—CHANGE FOREVER

Whether you are creating a healing response to illness, upgrading your moods or boosting energy, creativity requires a leap in awareness—that is, to be what you weren't before.

"When faced with the choice between changing and proving there's no need to do so, most people get busy on the proof..."
John Kenneth Galbraith

You are by nature a creative being. As a child you had a rich imagination. Your youthful present-moment awareness allowed you to quickly, without reason, form new perceptions and fun interpretations on an ongoing basis. A quantum leap—a paradigm shift—from one pattern of behavior to another without going through incremental steps has always advanced the world in art, music or science. Quantum leaps of creativity from prevailing patterns allowed William Shakespeare, Albert Einstein, Sir Robert Banting, Beethoven and the Beatles to change the world forever.

The health principles outlined in *The Path to Phenomenal Health* can provide you with the framework to achieve healthy vitality and wellness physically, mentally, emotionally and spiritually. I urge you to pay close attention to the principles outlined in this book and share them with the ones you love. Test-drive my Seven-Day Rejuvenation Plan and watch and feel your dynamic energy soar.

Sometimes we must all pursue noble efforts that perhaps Albert Einstein would approve. For eleven consecutive years, Einstein was nominated for a Nobel Prize only to be rejected. The theory of relativity proved to be too radical a concept for the Nobel committee. In 1921 he finally became a Nobel laureate. The committee directed Einstein not to mention relativity in his acceptance lecture. He did so anyway!

Remember, the consequences of your healthy choices will affect many more people than just yourself. You owe it to yourself, our global family and everyone you care about to achieve optimum vitality, emotional balance, spiritual maturity and healthy well-being. Your ability to handle adversity defines you. Your circumstances are not always ideal, but circumstances do not determine who you are. Reclaim your own freedom to determine who you are. Have great unshakable faith and most importantly, never give up hope.

Hope is the thing with feathers—
That perches in the soul—
And sings the tune without the words—
And never stops—at all—

Emily Dickinson

Part III

REVITALIZE

11

EAT IN TUNE WITH YOUR GENETIC CODE

HOW WELL DO YOU EAT?

Genetically we have evolved, but so have the ever-available processed, synthetic, refined foods. Can they fuel our magnificent 100 trillion cells? Today, genetics and lifestyle are colliding. To have your radiant vitality and brainpower operating at optimum, it is critical to fuel yourself with a diet true to your ancient genetic origin and makeup. You can:

- Reset your genetic code
- Lose weight permanently
- Achieve peak performance
- Enhance mental sharpness

The landscape of your brain and body, the actual architecture and intricate wiring, was formed by the seasonal foods available at the time. Roughly 99.9 percent of your genetic structure was formed even before the advent of agriculture ten thousand or so years ago.

The miraculous engineering, hardwiring and perfect performance of the body and mind were based on a genetic makeup that allowed our early ancestors to function as nature designed. Our ancestors grew and developed their digestion, absorption, distribution and elimination processes based on cell-friendly foods that were compatible, body ready, and readily abundant thousands of years before the advent of fast-food chains, junk food and late-night corner stores.

Remarkably, most people today fuel themselves with processed convenience foods, sweet-tasting foods, and chemically altered foods that are attractively and colorfully packaged. This "food-stuff" we now ingest has the unprecedented, stunning ability to be only one molecule away from being plastic. New miracle-age fast-food chains are booming with catchy advertising promises in a land where dairy is queen and burger is king.

So while our genetic makeup (genome) and origin have changed only 0.01 percent in the last ten thousand years, our lifestyle has changed 99 percent. Our hunter-gatherer ancestors were aerobically fit. They were virtually free of the chronic "lifestyle diseases" that cause 85 percent of all illness in North America today.

AN AWESOME BIOLOGICAL JOLT

Our shift from hunting and gathering to agriculture, and from the industrial revolution to industry, has drastically changed human nutrition with an extremely detrimental biological jolt, which in turn has promoted heart disease, cancer, stroke, depression, diabetes and a prevailing sense of drop-dead fatigue.

> Change the environment knowingly or unknowingly and the environment is guaranteed to change you. "Food-stuff"—the degraded foods of modern commerce—that are unfamiliar to your genes, brain and body, trigger serious intracellular communication breakdowns leading to daily power outages.

There is now a worrisome decrease in our consumption of lean, high-quality protein; very low-density complex carbohydrates, such as vegetables, greens, salads, spices and herbs; and moderate-density complex carbohydrates, such as fruits, berries and minimally processed grains. These cell-friendly foods contain a little naturally occurring sugar for a steady energy supply and a lot of life-supportive fiber, water, vitamins, minerals, antioxidants and phytonutrients.

THE ANCIENT DIET YOUR BRAIN AND BODY DEMAND

Your body and brain are organic structures. One hundred percent of the foods you feed to your cells determine their architectural structure, their optimum energy output potential, their ability to function and your daily rejuvenation potential.

Your body's hardwired network communication systems are based on the *available enzymes* found in vegetables, wild greens, nuts, seeds, roots, herbs, spices, fruits, sea vegetables and grass-fed, lean animals that your ancestors gathered or hunted.

Your biological ancestors instinctively learned to use *naturally protective antioxidants* from freshly gathered plants, such as wild greens, to protect their oxygen-based life processes. Their bodies also learned to use *naturally protective phytonutrients* from freshly gathered plants to protect and restore their cells, brains, vital energy, digestive tracts, organs and communication networks from daily wear-and-tear, plus eliminate ever-lurking bacteria, viruses, parasites, yeast overgrowth and carcinogens. Food always has been, and always will be, the best medicine.

BROCCOLI VERSUS ANTIBIOTICS

A study published in the *Proceedings of the National Academy of Sciences* explained that the phytonutrient found in broccoli, called sulforaphane, eradicated the stomach bacteria *H. pylori* 100 percent, while antibiotics were 80 percent effective. Johns Hopkins University researchers point out that some strains of *H. pylori* are up to 20 percent drug-resistant; *no* strain is resistant to sulforaphane. Only nature provides cell-friendly foods as medicine that support your ancient genetic makeup.

Our species, *Homo sapiens*, managed to evolve to meet the challenges of hungry predators and a hostile environment. We were, and are, the most complex physiological species and consequently we are the most vulnerable. Our modern-day eating patterns are counterproductive! In only fifty years, we have reached the point where we run our miraculous engineering on empty calories and troublesome nutrients that were never part of our genetic makeup or natural origin.

YOUR DAILY STRESSORS SEND FAULTY EATING SIGNALS TO YOUR GENES

Researchers at the University of California, San Francisco discovered that our drive for comfort foods is built in. Rats under chronic stress that were given the option of high-nutrition rat chow or a mixture of lard and sugar headed for the latter every time. And their choice actually did lower their stress-hormone levels.

In terms of evolution, the response makes sense: If a hungry predator is chasing us, easily digested and high-caloric foods like fat and sugar give us quick fuel for a speedy escape. "In a sense," explains Norman Pecoraro, PhD, co-author of this study, "it's a survival appetite," but only temporarily. In the long run, Dr. Pecoraro quickly adds, opting for fat and sugar will cause you to tip your energy balance negatively. Too much caffeine only increases the jitters. Alcohol lifts and then drops spirits, and hunger and thirst are themselves stressful. Eating regular meals and snacks throughout the day of high-fiber, slowly digested, healthy, cell-friendly foods keeps your blood sugar even, which keeps your energy and mood boosted.

MICROWAVING IS NOT CELL-FRIENDLY

The *Journal of the Science of Food and Agriculture* studied the effects of various cooking methods and the reduction of nutritional value.

All cooking breaks down the nutritional values of food to certain degrees.

Microwaving, used in 91.3 percent of North American households, destroys 97 percent of the life-saving antioxidants and between 74 and 87 percent of the healthful polyphenols. Microwaving is the worst depleter of nutrients.

Lightly steaming food maintained the highest nutritional value and maximized flavor—followed by pressure cooking and boiling.

NATURE'S SUPERCRITICAL CELL-FRIENDLY FOODS

Ten Tips to Eating Smart for Robust Energy and Good Moods

The recipe for smart eating—to give your 100 trillion cells remarkable energy and vitality with body-ready nutrition—is to eat in harmony with your long-standing genetic predisposition to food.

1. Make colorful fresh fruits, berries, vegetables, including crisp salads, herbs, and spices like garlic and turmeric, and a diverse variety of greens and sea vegetables (like Nova Scotia dulse) the major part of your daily diet. Do not eat any extra calories you do not need.
2. Eat raw foods at each meal, such as nuts, seeds, salads, sprouts or veggie sticks.
3. Eat unsalted nuts and seeds, especially almonds, walnuts, pumpkin seeds, flax seeds, hemp seeds, sesame seeds and six macadamia nuts daily for omega-7 fats.
4. Eat plenty of fatty cold-water fish, primarily anchovies, sardines, mackerel and salmon. For long-chain omega-3 essential fatty acids, take fish oil capsules derived from anchovies, sardines and mackerel for preformed and biologically active "mood smart" EPA and "brain smart" DHA fats every day.
5. Eat wild game, and lean free-range meats and poultry without the skin and subcutaneous fat. Eat 20 to 30 grams of lean animal-based or lean plant-based protein at each meal.

   Eat unsalted beans and legumes of all types, such as lentils, soybeans, edamame, split peas, chick peas or their by-products, such as extra-firm tofu, tempeh, miso, natto and seitan.

   A soy constituent called lunasin increases the activity of cancer-suppressing genes and repairs damaged DNA in men's prostate cells.
6. Omit processed, convenient, refined foods full of taste-enhancing chemicals, spoilage retardants, synthetic colors, preservatives, and so few critical vitamins, minerals, antioxidants or phytonutrients. They are high-calorie, low-nutrient foods. Limit your use of sugar, added fructose, high-fructose corn syrup, artificial sweeteners and salt. Stevia is a good, safe sweetener.
7. Drink lots of fresh, clean water. Daily drink 2 to 4 cups of organic green or matcha tea.

8. Daily, use omega-9 extra-virgin olive oil. Grind 2 tablespoons of high-lignan flax seeds in a coffee grinder and add to your breakfast protein shake for cancer protection. Add 2 tablespoons of ground sesame seeds if you need an immune boost.

   Restrict omega-6 fats, especially corn oil and vegetable oils like sunflower and safflower, and limit even flax seed oil since these oils can cause excessive inflammation in your body, potentially leading to heart disease and cancer. Dr. Anna J. Duffield-Lillico of the Sloan-Kettering Cancer Center proved that oxidative metabolism of linoleic acids contributes to the formation of cancerous colon tumors.

   Do use unsalted organic butter in moderation (1 to 2 tablespoons per day).

   Use 1 to 2 tablespoons daily of virgin coconut oil, made only from fresh coconuts, not copras (dried coconuts). Coconut oil has the consistency of soft butter, can substitute for butter and is rich in lauric acid, which is known to be antiviral, antibacterial and antifungal.

   Avoid trans fats and acrylamides in fried foods, fast foods, commercial bakery goods and in any processed foods containing hydrogenated or semi-hydrogenated fats or oils. These fats are unfamiliar to your body and brain—they trigger serious cellular communication malfunctions.
9. Daily use food-based vitamin/mineral supplements, antioxidant spices, medicinal herbs, herbal teas, sea vegetables and today's version of wild greens, an extra-energy "green drink" because you need a supplemental power shift to imitate your ancestors' nutrient-rich diet.
10. Have a daily glass of fresh vegetable juice emphasizing gene-supportive herbs and spices.

MY FAVORITE VEGETABLE JUICE RECIPE, FROM MY GRANDMA NANA MARIE

- 2 medium-sized carrots (because of their high sugar content)
- ½ small red beet

- Large piece of fresh ginger, chopped (1 tablespoon)
- 1 stalk of celery with leaves
- 6 stems of each: watercress, cilantro and parsley
- Juice of ½ lemon
- ½ yellow or orange pepper
- 1 small red tomato

Optional

- 1 clove of garlic and/or a dash of any salt-free, non-irradiated herbal seasoning
- Dash of cayenne pepper or curry or turmeric

FATIGUE REMEDY—EAT A CELL-FRIENDLY DIET

Each one of your cells is part of the intricate assembly line of your body. Remember, *every minute, 200 million new cells are renewed and revitalized in your body. This is a total of 300 billion new cells a day*. Your cells have no part in your food selection. They have no ability to choose. They must do the best they can with what is available, whether the food is synthetic or natural. They have only an inherited ability to sort through the immediate supply, good or bad. Each time you eat, your cells jump up and get to work to sort and absorb. They never ease up. To maintain well-being, cells require a constant supply of steady energy.

Cells can become exhausted trying to find critical nutrients in French fries, colas, diet pops, potato chips or processed foods that are no longer whole foods. Many of the necessary parts of these foods are missing because of refining and processing.

THREE BALANCED MEALS AND TWO SNACKS PER DAY FOR SUPERIOR ENERGY, STAMINA AND MOOD

The Harvard Newsletter reported that the average North American, in his or her lifetime, eats 66,000 pounds of food or "food-stuff." This is the approximate weight of eight mature elephants. *When* you eat your food is just as critically important as *what* you eat.

Neurocognitive researcher and author of *Optimum Sports Nutrition* Dr. Michael Colgan states that "You need to eat three calorically balanced, nutrient-dense meals and two snacks a day." He points out that skipping a meal because you are in a rush, or while you are trying to juggle a heavy schedule, or are multi-tasking, or intentionally cutting back on calories is totally unproductive. It backfires on you, causing you to literally store more fat.

Our biological ancestors, whose gene expressions we have inherited, lived by the seasonal availability of food, which Canadian endocrinologist Dr. Hans Selye called "feast or famine." He explains: "When we skip a meal, this causes the body enormous stress." The body interprets a skipped meal as a sign of pending famine and instinctively, just like our biological ancestors' genes learned to do, we store extra fat from our next meal as a future energy resource to see us through the next life-threatening famine.

A survey of the eating habits of nearly fifteen thousand residents of Norfolk, England, aged forty-five to seventy-five, found that people who ate three meals and two snacks a day had an average cholesterol level that was 5 percent lower than the ones who ate one or two meals a day. This study, reported in the *British Medical Journal,* has researchers speculating that we store more of the fat when we gorge than when we eat or graze more regularly.

DO NOT EAT AFTER 8:00 P.M.

Eating shortly before sleeping will raise insulin levels, which prevent melatonin from spiking. Because of late-night eating habits, poor sleep patterns and accumulated sleep debt, peak nighttime melatonin levels of most people sixty-five or older are only 30 to 40 picograms per milliliter of blood, whereas a twenty-five-year-old secretes 100 to 2,000 picograms per milliliter of blood at night. Melatonin is also your system-wide, natural anticancer hormone. Do not let it dwindle on you.

THE ANCIENT EATING PATTERN YOUR BRAIN AND BODY DEMAND

7:00 a.m. a well-balanced breakfast

10:00 a.m. a pre-planned snack

noon a well-balanced lunch

3:00 p.m. a pre-planned snack

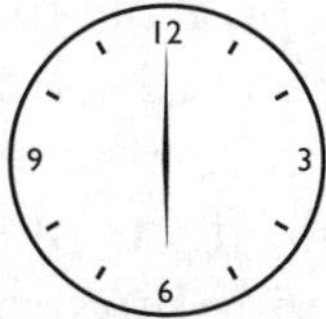

6:00 p.m. a well-balanced supper

EATING BALANCED MEALS

Begin thinking of food in terms of its three major categories: protein, carbohydrates and fats. These three are the only essential foods to eat. Only then can you easily master the basic rules for controlling another hormone called insulin. Insulin is the primary factor in gaining or losing excess body fat, in preventing type II diabetes and for storing the glucose (sugar molecule) broken down from eating carbohydrates in your trillions of energy-producing mitochondria.

Glucose is the primary fuel, the control rod, in your nuclear energy reactor, the mitochondria. Insulin is a storage hormone and it literally pushes or "ushers" glucose and protein into your cells to be used as fuel and structure.

Controlling neurotransmitters and hormones may seem confusing and difficult at first. The truth is that you don't really need to understand all the intricate workings of your hormone system to get the balanced level of hormones that your body needs. All you have to do is follow the very basic dietary steps I am outlining and make them a habit!

TOTAL GLYCEMIC LOAD: NUTRITIONAL NEUROSCIENCE

Your mind-body requires homeostasis (metabolic balance), which means your blood sugar or energy supply stays constant, as do your vital control-program hormones, such as glucagon, insulin, thyroid hormones, estrogen and testosterone, so you do not experience mood swings and depressive letdowns.

Low-glycemic index foods like vegetables, salads and fruit provide energy in a slow- and sustained-release form, reducing hunger and facilitating the smooth use and storage of calories. It is very difficult to over-consume low-density carbohydrates such as salads, vegetables and fruit because of their very high fiber, water, vitamin and mineral levels. They also slow sugar's rate of entry into the bloodstream, thereby maintaining the best possible insulin control.

High-glycemic index foods like bagels, white rice or French bread provoke strong insulin responses, increasing the exposure of your body to the harmful effects of excess insulin. These high-glycemic index foods do provide bursts of energy, but are generally followed by hunger, fatigue, restlessness, severe mood swings and depleted energy, and cause further bingeing and craving cycles.

This does not mean high-glycemic index foods are all bad and low-glycemic index foods are all good. It is important to keep the total glycemic load low at each meal.

You must consider that the proportion of high-glycemic index foods in the diet is an important variable when evaluating health risks. As an example, 1 cup of cooked pasta has the same amount of carbohydrates as 12 cups of broccoli. At any given meal, keep the *total glycemic load* low. The total glycemic load is the average glycemic index of all the foods you eat at a meal or snack.

Eating protein causes the release of the hormone glucagon, which is a counter-regulatory hormone, an antidote that keeps insulin levels in check and normalizes blood sugar by raising or lowering it as needed. Glucagon delivers glucose to your brain. Most people are not aware that high blood sugar and elevated insulin have serious implications for increased degenerative brain diseases, including Alzheimer's. In Alzheimer's there are abnormalities in how the brain metabolizes glucose (sugar), resulting in the overproduction of nerve damage, silent inflammation and free radicals and the formation of neurofibrillary tangles and gooey beta amyloid protein clusters that kill off brain cells.

Each meal should have a perfect balance of the protein-to-carbohydrate ratio, which means you have a perfect balance of glucagon to insulin—a perfectly balanced intracellular communication system for robust body energy and smart, revitalized brainpower. If you keep blood insulin levels low, you burn body fat for energy and lose weight naturally.

VISUALLY DIVIDE YOUR PLATE INTO THIRDS

The Protein-to-Carbohydrate Ratio

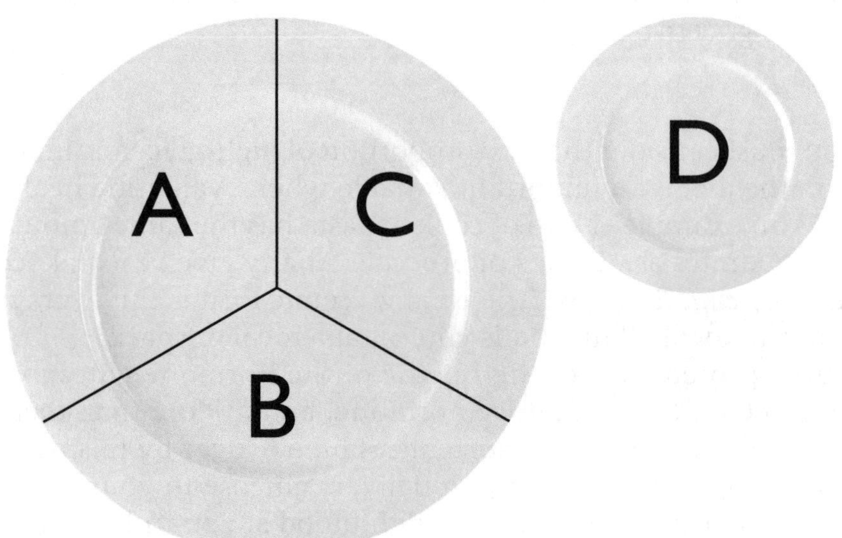

A = lean protein 20-25 grams per meal for women
30-35 grams per meal for men
15-20 grams per meal for children
lean, animal-based source: size and thickness of your palm
plant-based source: 2 cups of vegetable protein

B = colorful, crunchy-tender *vegetables* that are very low-density carbohydrates

C = colorful, crispy *salad* with olive oil

D = side dish—baked *yam, sweet potato* or *whole grain rice*

Three Quick Ways to Lower a Meal's Total Glycemic Load

When the total glycemic load of a meal is high, it sends a signal to your body to produce lipogenic enzymes, such as lipoprotein lipase, in abundance, which turn on fat cells to expand and store body fuel.

When the total glycemic load of a meal or snack is low, your fat cells receive a signal to produce lipolytic enzymes like hormone-sensitive lipase to turn off fat cells from a fat-storage mode and to actively begin to burn body fat as energy.

FIRST: Eat 20 to 30 grams of lean protein at every meal and eat it first.

SECOND: Always eat fresh colorful vegetables as part of your meals. Vegetables and salad are made up of both soluble and insoluble fibers that slow down the rate at which glucose enters your bloodstream. You need a minimum of 35 grams of fiber a day—my recommendations in this book will ensure that you receive 40 grams.

THIRD: Liberally sprinkle fresh lemon juice, apple cider vinegar or cinnamon on, or in, your food and protein shakes and you lower the glycemic value of the meal by an average of 30 percent, according to the *American Journal of Clinical Nutrition*.

EAT IN TUNE WITH YOUR GENETIC CODE

These steps are scientifically sound and allow you to properly adjust and alter your neurotransmitters, neuropeptides and hormones on a twenty-four-hour on-call dedicated line that will keep your brain, mind, emotions, enthusiasm, creativity and optimum energy in peak condition for a bright future.

Remember: just follow the common sense approach of your ancestors. Use balance, variety and moderation at each meal and snack.

Balance your plate with the proper variety of lean proteins, both colorful vegetable and salad carbohydrates, and essential fats at your three meals. Moderation tells us never to eat too many calories in one meal or snack. At every meal, visually divide your plate into three portions. Now add a cell-friendly, natural, low-glycemic, complex carbohydrate source as a condiment. Colorful plant foods and lean protein have marvelous capabilities to balance your insulin and glucagon blood levels, allowing you to maintain robust energy and brainpower throughout the day.

TWO FORGOTTEN VITAMINS—THE FUTURE OF DISEASE PREVENTION AND STRONG BONES

Vitamin D: The *American Journal of Medicine*, as well as William B. Grant, PhD, one of the top vitamin D researchers in the world, states that 80 to 90 percent of North Americans are chronically deficient in vitamin D. Low levels of vitamin D contribute to cancer, osteoporosis, multiple sclerosis, arthritis and depression.

Jennifer Wider, MD, from the Society for Women's Health Research, emphasizes that vitamin D works in the intestines to escort calcium into the bloodstream and also in the kidneys to help absorb calcium that would otherwise be excreted. Vitamin D enhances the ability of calcium to be absorbed into the osteoblast cells of bones.

Haojie Li, MD, PhD, of Harvard University, found that high-plasma vitamin D levels protect against prostate cancer. The *Journal of the National Cancer Institute* reported in 2005 that increased, prudent sun exposure led to increased survivability of cancer patients. The Karolinska Institute in Sweden, in 2005, reduced non-Hodgkin's lymphoma by 40 percent with sun exposure. The *Journal of the National Cancer Institute* published research on vitamin D's role in preventing colon cancer and, when combined with calcium, the anticancer effect was even greater. Most people do not know they are depleted in vitamin D because that has become their normal state. There are two blood tests your physician can use to measure your vitamin D levels—1,25(OH)D and 25(OH)D. Request the 25(OH)D, as it is a better marker of overall vitamin D status.

Sunlight is every bit as central to your health and well-being as proper nutrition, deep breathing to oxygenate tissues, clean water, deep sleep and exercise. Dr. Michael Holick, director of the Vitamin D Skin and Bone Research Lab at Boston University, and biochemist Reinhold Viet, PhD, of the University of Toronto, tell us to supplement with vitamin D3 during sunless months. Use safe levels of 400 to 1,000 International Units (IU) per day on those grey days of winter, or throughout the year if you would rather avoid the necessary ten minutes a day of direct "safe sun" void of sunscreen.

Vitamin K: Vitamin K1, or phylloquinone, is found in any green vegetable containing the green pigment chlorophyll and its water-soluble derivative, chlorophyllin. Vitamin K1, in the presence of "friendly" bacteria in the intestines, is converted into the more biologically active form called K2, or memaquinones. K2 is found in egg yolk, butter and fermented soy foods. K2 helps the body make and activate two critical proteins, osteocalcin and matrix G1a, in a biochemical process called gamma-carboxylation. Osteocalcin and matrix Gla are calcium-binding proteins, absolutely essential to guide calcium into the osteoblast cells of bones, make strong bone tissues and prevent osteoporosis.

If you do not have sufficient vitamin K2 status, calcium may deposit in soft tissues like arteries, your heart and your brain and cause strokes, heart attacks, Alzheimer's and dementia. Vitamin K2 simultaneously reduces the risk of osteoporosis, arteriosclerosis and memory loss. The journal *Nutrition* quotes the Rotterdam Study of 4,983 men and women, from 1990 until 2002, that proves vitamin K2 helps to protect against heart disease and memory loss. The September 2003 *International Journal of Oncology* revealed that treating lung cancer patients with vitamin K2 slowed the growth of cancer cells. Main message: eat lots of deep green vegetables, parsley, cilantro, watercress, culinary herbs and "green drinks" daily. If you are on an anticoagulant drug like Coumadin, check with your physician before you overconsume vitamin K2 because it has a blood-thinning effect.

A CELL-FRIENDLY HEALTH BOOSTER: WATER

Researchers at the Fred Hutchinson Research Center in Seattle found that women who drank two glasses of water a day had nearly twice the risk of colon cancer as women who drank four glasses per day. And what makes the data particularly convincing is that the women in the study who drank eight or more glasses of water per day had less than half the risk of those who drank only four glasses. Even more striking is the association of increased water intake and reduced risk of other types of cancer. In one study, the women who drank the most water were 80 percent less likely to develop bladder cancer than women who drank the least.

REMEMBER THIS IRREFUTABLE FACT

The absence of a sense of thirst is not a reliable indicator of the need for water. Drink your eight glasses every day, whether you are thirsty or not. Do not wait for thirst signals; prehydrate rather than rehydrate. Often you misinterpret thirst signals as hunger signs and eat unnecessary calories when you really should be drinking revitalizing water.

Cells Organize Water in Multilayered Structures

The human body and mind are a hologram. "Living water" from fruits and vegetables organizes itself in layers and patterns in each cell to promote high-quality intracellular communication. Water does not just fill a space; water has an organizational skill that has stunned veteran researchers.

An ancient biological dance happens to water once it enters the cells of your body. The molecules of water you drink from the tap, bottle or spring are arranged in random clusters. Once these water molecules find their way into your 100 trillion cells, however, they become highly organized. Molecular biologists at Rice University and the University of California have confirmed that intracellular water is very different from other forms of water. Organized water in cells is genetically designed to direct the flow of enzymes and cell-signalling communication pathways.

Water appears to exist within the cell in a complex, multilayered, organized structure. Imagine that the water in your glass is like a container of alphabetical letters all mixed up. After you drink it, if you looked inside the cell with a high-resonance microscope, you would see words, sentences and paragraphs called clustering. Eat lots of fresh vegetables, salads and ripe fruit that contain organic "living water" that has already organized itself into the clusters—or words—your cells recognize.

Your skin is 80 percent water. The most important cosmetic help or nutritional support you can give yourself that will promote a clear, smooth, radiant complexion is to drink clean, pure water throughout the day.

One of water's most important functions is to maintain and influence protein structure, thus maintaining the intimate connection with anabolic metabolism. In the past, researchers merely looked for the presence or absence of water, but a whole new world of biophysics has started to unfold. Drs. G. Alfred Gilman and Martin Rodbell won a Nobel Prize for their work with protein folding and specifically for describing the role that proteins play in intracellular communication. Amazingly, it has been shown that a cluster of organized water exists within these protein molecules. In fact, Dr. Julia Goodfellow at Birbeck College in London has shown that it is the interaction of structured water with other molecules that instructs the protein to fold and perform its strategic function. Surprisingly, water is responsible for maintaining the muscle-to-fat ratio. An obese man may have a water content of approximately 43 percent, whereas a lean man of the same age can have a water content of 65 percent or more. Likewise, the water content of an average forty-five-year-old man is 67 percent, but by age seventy, this decreases to approximately 45 percent. Clearly, the ability to daily restore optimum levels of water to your biological system will have profound effects on the entire mind-body connection and circuitry.

LESSONS FROM TRADITIONAL DIETS AND LIFESTYLES

In the Hunza Valley in Pakistan, in the Caucasus mountains in the former Soviet Union, in the Mediterranean area, and in the Andes mountains in South America, there are areas where people routinely live to be one hundred years of age or more. These people are energetic, lean and exceedingly healthy. The secret to their longevity, exceptional vitality and well-being lies in a healthy lifestyle, natural stress reduction and the type of diet I recommend to you. Some traditions we can accept and some we have to adjust and transform with modern-day adaptation.

Lessons from the Okinawan Diet and Lifestyle

There is modern documentation on the healthiest, most energetic and longest living people on the earth—those on the Japanese islands of Okinawa. According to the conclusions of the prominent researchers Drs. Bradley Wilcox, Craig Wilcox and Makoto Suzuki, these people are the healthiest and most energetic in the world. The many Okinawans who have lived one hundred years or more have been studied for twenty-five years. The study revealed that Okinawans are at a much lower risk than other people, including other Japanese, for age-related degenerative illnesses including heart disease, stroke, mental dementia, diabetes and almost all types of cancer. They are lean, healthy people virtually free of obesity.

Okinawans eat a low-calorie diet of about 1,500 to 1,800 calories per day. This diet is extremely low in salt, trans fatty acids, sugar and processed foods, but very high in vegetables, fruit and other plant foods, soy products like natto and miso, and freshly ground flax seed. They eat fish rich in EPA and DHA omega-3 essential fatty acids. They stir-fry their foods lightly in canola oil, rich in omega-9 and omega-6 fats, from the indigenous rapeseed plant. Okinawans eat, on average, ten to twenty servings a day of fresh vegetables and fruit. They are also very physically active with gardening, walking, even-paced working and participating in traditional dance and Tai Chi. These activities are potent stress-alert busters. They eat, on average, 40 grams of fiber every day. It is interesting to note that they average nine hours of sleep every night.

Lessons from the Mediterranean Diet and Lifestyle

The best modern-day example of a traditional diet that can promote vitality and wellness and prevent heart disease, cancer, stroke, diabetes and weight gain comes from the Mediterranean region, including southern Italy, Spain, Portugal, southern France, Greece and the Greek island of Crete. What is so great about these people's diet?

Salads, vegetables, beans, whole grains and fruit are extremely popular. Beans include chick peas, lentils, split peas and fava beans. The most commonly eaten whole grains are polenta, couscous, bulgar, rice and wheat. Lean meat such as lamb, chicken and beef are eaten in small portions. Aside from a small amount of natural cheese and butter, milk products are not generally part of the Mediterranean diet. Interestingly, these people have a lower incidence of osteoporosis than we do in North America, where we consume large amounts of dairy products.

Fresh fruit is a typical dessert and the Mediterranean diet contains very few processed foods. Fresh fruits, which include berries, grapes, figs, prunes, apricots, melons, lemons, tangerines and oranges, are the most commonly consumed fruits. Dry red wine, high in polyphenols, is consumed in small amounts with meals. The diet features lots of herbs and spices, including garlic, parsley, cilantro, hot peppers, basil, bay leaf, oregano, rosemary, mint, dill, thyme and spices like turmeric, cloves, ginger, garlic and cinnamon, which are all known and proven to inhibit cancer cell colonies from initiating or proliferating. These vegetables, herbs and spices promote immune health and both Phase I and Phase II detoxification enzymes. A growing body of research indicates that many herbs and spices can help you prevent cancer. Curcumin, the yellow pigment in turmeric, is a new darling among anticancer researchers and has been proven to prevent and treat Alzheimer's disease. Rosemary and ginger are COX-2 inhibitors that block enzymes, preventing cancer cells from growing. Garlic, oregano and basil kill viruses and bacteria. Use raw garlic in salads daily as it helps to prevent cancer.

The Mediterranean diet includes almost 30 percent of the calories as fat. But that is really not high, considering the quality of the fats, which are in the form of omega-3, omega-6 and omega-9. They get EPA and DHA, omega-3 fats, from eating fish like sardines, anchovies, tuna and salmon. They get omega-9 monounsaturated fat from olive oil, which decreases bad LDL cholesterol and raises good HDL cholesterol. They eat omega-3 and omega-6 fats in avocados, flax seeds, walnuts, sunflower seeds and the wild salad green purslane. They eat on average 40 grams of fiber daily. The Mediterranean people have developed wonderful stress busters, such as an afternoon nap, eating slowly and savoring their meals, close family ties, joyful ethnic dancing and robust happy singing. Once again, it is interesting to note that the Mediterraneans themselves also average nine hours of sleep a night.

12

BEYOND CLEANSING: DAILY DETOX

YOUR FILTERS MAY NEED CLEANING

Cellular detoxification is a powerful anabolic, therapeutic tool you must keep handy in your genetic toolbox. The advances made in research in this information age have enabled us to immediately alter our lifestyle and diet for enhanced brainpower and more dynamic energy.

The bottom line is that to remain at peak performance levels, you need to protect your cells from the toxic by-products of a modern technological society. If you want to eliminate the toxins you daily breathe, drink and eat, knowingly or unknowingly, you need to consider detoxification.

AN IRREFUTABLE FACT

The average person has 6 pounds of putrifying waste lining the intestinal walls by the age of twenty-four.

Detoxification is a metabolic cleansing—cleaning chemicals and toxic substances from the body before they harm your cells. Left to their own, these exotoxins (*exo-* means from outside the body) are very harmful.

Your body uses a one-two punch to eliminate exotoxins like alcohol, pesticides, preservatives, insidious trans fats and chemical pollutants.

For example, the more your car or truck is neglected, the more gunk builds up in and around the motor, impairing the motor's efficiency and longevity. You must change the oil filter and air filter in your vehicle's motor. You also clean vacuum cleaner bags and furnace, air conditioner and clothes dryer filters. The more you clean, restore, rebuild or renew your body's filters, the less intracellular trash and gunk will accumulate in your 100 trillion cells, and the longer and healthier you will live.

EXOTOXINS AND ENDOTOXINS

Your body and cells are incredibly adaptable to positive changes, but we live in a toxic world and put constant pressure on them. Toxins come from car fumes, pesticides, additives, and chemicals blown from industrial smoke stacks hundreds of miles away. They are in tobacco, alcohol, coffee, French fries, donuts, prescription drugs and over-the-counter drugs, as well as recreational drugs. They all leave toxic residues in your cells.

Your intestines host over four hundred species of microorganisms, "friendly" bacteria, weighing an astonishing 2 full kilos.

Even plants have toxins in them, as do animals fed food containing growth hormones, antibiotics and other animal parts. As if this weren't enough, your body produces endotoxins (*endo-* means inside), the waste by-products of your own cellular metabolism.

Although your body has been designed with several built-in filtration systems, even these systems become overloaded in today's toxic environment. Some of these exo- and endotoxins are water-soluble, and your body excretes them in your urine or stool. Some are fat-soluble and accumulate in fatty tissues where they become hard to cleanse and eliminate.

If you are very stressed, tired, eating poorly, underexercising or overexercising, or suffering from sleep debt, your body may not have the extra energy to clean its own filters efficiently and in a timely manner. Exotoxins and endotoxins are cumulative, adding to the toxic accumulated overload we call illness or disease. Like other biochemical breakdowns, toxins build up insidiously and without symptoms all life long until they are finally manifested in illness.

To survive well in a toxic world, you need to eliminate these toxins from sensitive cells every day before the cells are damaged.

YOUR FOUR KEY FILTRATION SYSTEMS

Filter 1: Your Liver. A healthy liver filters out and transforms both exotoxins and endotoxins that have entered your bloodstream into harmless intermediates that are eventually excreted in your sweat, urine and stool.

Filter 2: Your Intestines. The intestines expel toxins and microorganisms quickly through regular bowel movements. It is therefore important to have three bowel movements a day. The intestines, when in a healthy state, are full of "friendly" probiotic bacteria that confront and destroy toxins. Healthy intestinal walls act as an effective barrier that prevents toxins or toxic by-products from leaking back into the bloodstream while they move through the intestines to be expelled.

Filter 3: Your Kidneys. The kidneys' primary job is to take water-soluble toxins, render them harmless and expel them through urine.

Filter 4: Your Skin. The 6 pounds of skin on your body is an excellent filter that releases toxins out of its pores. After a hot day's work, a hard, sweaty workout or a sauna, your skin has the strong odor of toxin release.

Pain relievers such as aspirin may be band-aids masking accumulating toxins that require a detox.

HOW TO FLOURISH AND BE WELL IN A TOXIC WORLD

Of all the filtering and detoxification that goes on automatically in your body daily, most of it goes on in your liver. The liver takes exotoxins and endotoxins and transforms them into intermediate substances that can easily be excreted. This process, called biotransformation, happens in a two-phase process.

In Phase I, a large family of enzymes, called the cytochrome P450 system, transforms the toxins into metabolites. In Phase II these transformed metabolites are made water-soluble. Then they are attached to a transporter molecule, such as glutathione, and eliminated in the urine, stool or through perspiration. Unfortunately, if the transformation enzyme process of Phase I falters or is sluggish, the metabolites remain in Phase I form and are still extremely toxic. This process is called bioactivation of toxins. These bioactivated toxins start to autointoxicate—that is, they leak back into your bloodstream. This causes the body to go into toxic overload. This is why people feel worse in the initial stages of an improperly planned fast or detox and can break out in rashes or pimples.

SUPPORT YOUR DETOX WITH A CELL-FRIENDLY DIET

My grandmother would fast for two weeks each spring and fall on water and fruit or vegetable juices to clean toxins out of her body. For many years I did the very same thing, but a study published in the *Annual Review of Nutrition* demonstrated that fasting can concentrate toxins, actually causing them to *stick and stall* in Phase I detox processes. Fasting slows down the metabolic rate of Phase I. This research demonstrated that the cytochrome P450 mixed-function oxidase family of enzymes operates in eight separate Phase II processes and needs constant refuelling from protein to work efficiently. Fasting did the opposite; it reduced protein intake. Furthermore, research now shows that high carbohydrate intake impairs and reduces the ability of the P450 enzymes to work. Fasting on juices is counterproductive, raising blood glucose levels and making P450 enzymes less effective.

"If the liver can't use the Phase II pathways, bioactivated intermediates can accumulate and be more harmful to the body than if no detoxification had taken place at all."

Marianne Leblanc, MD, Optima Health Solutions, Vancouver

PHASE I AND PHASE II LIVER DETOXIFICATION PATHWAYS

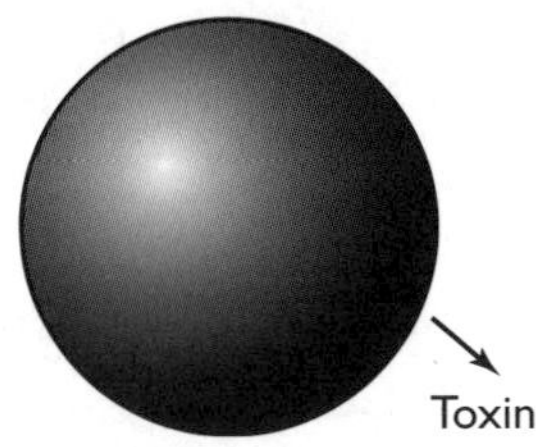

(A) Exotoxins and endotoxins enter your bloodstream and are taken to the liver.

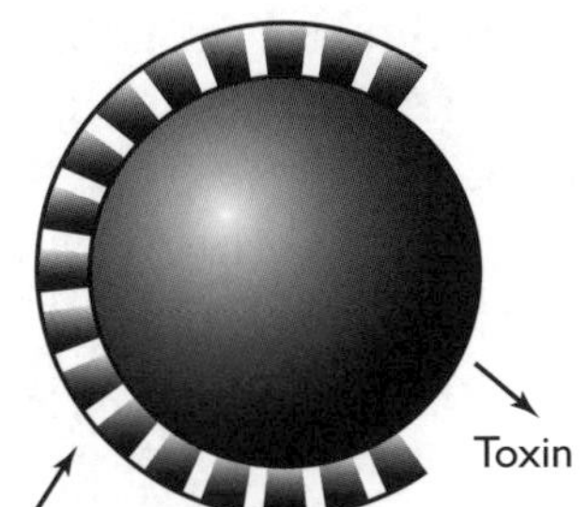

(B) The toxins are acted on by Phase I detoxification enzymes and have an oxygen molecule attached to them. The toxin is altered by the cytochrome P450 family of enzymes to a water-soluble biotransformed intermediate.

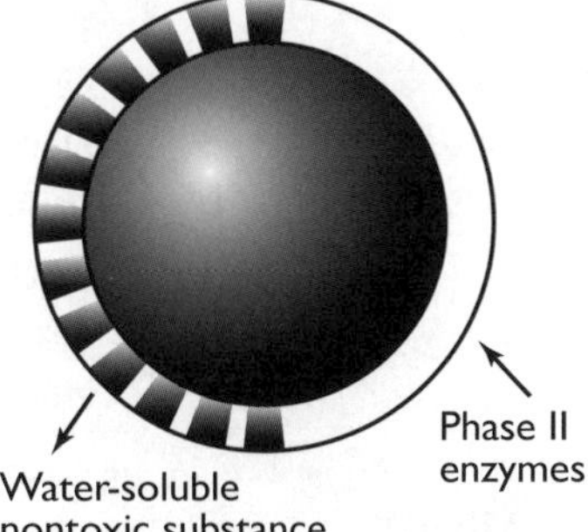

(C) If the diet is high in phytonutrients, then Phase II detoxification enzymes are activated by Nrf2 proteins that neutralize the toxin, convert it, then attach the toxin to a large carrier molecule like glutathione, which carries it out of the cell and eliminates it from the body as a water-soluble nontoxic substance.

Protein, vitamin C, antioxidants, phytonutrients such as silymarin (which is an extract of the herb milk thistle), calcium D-glutarate, indole-3-carbinol, the amino acids taurine and L-glutamine, non-dairy probiotic cultures, and both organic flax seed lignans and rice bran are needed by Phase I and Phase II enzyme systems to promote optimum detoxification.

The phytonutrients indole-3-carbinol and calcium D-glutarate from broccoli or any of the other cruciferous vegetables can increase the liver's ability to function in Phase II biotransformations by helping the liver convert chemicals that might be cancer-producing into non-toxic intermediates that can be excreted safely. Phytonutrients and active ingredients in both herbs and spices—including flavones and flavonols in dandelion root; proanthocyanidins in red wine, green tea, grape seed and skin extract; indoles from kale and artichoke leaf extract; lycopene from tomatoes; quercetin from citrus bioflavonoids; polysaccharides from spirulina, chlorella and Nova Scotia dulse; and chlorophyll from wheat grass, just to name a few, *are major therapeutic liver supporters*. They prevent toxins from attacking the liver and support healthy liver function.

USE A FOOD SUPPLEMENT FOR DAILY METABOLIC DETOXIFICATION

Food supplements are simple living solutions in a complex world that will help you quickly boost internal detoxification and rejuvenate powerful, deep, full body cleansing in each one of your 100 trillion cells.

Superior Metabolic Detoxification—Today!

Immediately boost your environmental toxin defenses and full body deep cleansing with the breakthrough, all natural, "perfect cleansing food" *greens+ daily detox*.

This is the first comprehensive nutritional support for Phase I and Phase II detoxification pathways to transform exotoxins (xenobiotics), the foreign chemicals, and endotoxins, the daily natural biological waste, into easily excreted, water-soluble compounds rather than into toxic fat-soluble compounds that accumulate and are difficult to eliminate, leading to toxic overload, weight gain, indigestion, malabsorption of critical nutrients, declining energy levels and eventual illness.

greens+ daily detox does several important things: (1) it promotes healthy gastrointestinal ecology, cleansing the small intestinal tract and the colon with fiber that has a gentle sweeping action; (2) it re-introduces viable friendly probiotic cultures all along the intestinal tract; (3) it supports superior digestion and enhanced absorption of nutrients; (4) it deeply and safely cleanses and detoxifies the liver, kidneys, blood and skin; and (5) it confronts, immobilizes and eliminates toxins in the digestive tract and supports the complex, multi-faceted process of biotransformation of accumulated environmental toxins by supporting both Phase I and Phase II detoxification systems.

To support detoxification and deep cleansing of your liver, kidneys, blood and skin, this formula is made with the finest, comprehensive, unique blend of binding nutrients, integrated natural herbs, potent antioxidants, critical amino acids and the most nourishing, chlorophyll-rich, cell-friendly foods available to powerfully initiate and support optimum Phase I and Phase II enzyme detoxification pathways. This will ensure that you are on the right track to having a long, happy, disease-free life.

greens+ daily detox

It is designed to support daily deep cleansing and metabolic detoxification, or conditions that may be associated with environmental pollution, accumulated toxins and cellular metabolic toxicity:

- irritability, anger, tension (especially after periods of emotional or chemical stress)
- migraine headaches or drop-dead fatigue
- an overly sensitive stomach
- fibromyalgia
- chronic fatigue syndrome
- food allergies and intolerances, such as gluten or milk sensitivities
- alcohol and chemical dependency

- candida infections
- chemical or environmental sensitivities
- irritable bowel syndrome (IBS)
- a reduced sense of overall mental or physical well-being
- for people with amalgam fillings; those with maldigestion and malabsorption, flatulence and bloating; "foggy mind" syndrome or lack of concentration; and those who commute to and from work in heavy traffic

THE DETOXIFICATION AND REJUVENATION PROGRAM: MANAGING TOXINS FROM WITHIN

Surprisingly, disease states generally originate in our late teens and early twenties, with function slowly deteriorating. Symptoms begin to increase from accumulated toxins. Most illnesses are related to problems of the digestive, liver and intestinal detoxification systems and you need to begin to detoxify daily or weekly. Dr. Hans Selye, MD, who was a pioneer in the study of stress, believed that modern people lose their ability to eliminate toxins when the body is in a state of continued stress. He described most people as having sluggish digestion and compromised liver function that impairs efficient, daily detoxification, and elimination of toxins, which Jean-Yves Dionne, a master pharmacist and nutritional researcher from Montreal, calls "the walking-wounded-syndrome." Long-term accumulation of environmental toxins burdens the liver and immune system, impairs energy production, destroys intestinal linings and causes headaches, indigestion, irritability and fatigue.

Nutritional Genomics

Raymond Rodriguez, who heads the Center of Excellence in Nutritional Genomics at the University of California, Davies, believes that in coming years doctors will be able to take genetic profiles of their patients, identify specific diseases for which they are at risk and create customized nutritional plans. His work is based on the interplay of nutrition and genes, another variation of mind-body medicine.

I am personally interested in his work because he examines Phase I and Phase II detoxification pathways. It is desirable to have a balance of the two enzyme phases, but some people have a variant gene that speeds up Phase I enzymes, so they form carcinogens faster than Phase II enzymes can get rid of them. This gene is found in 28 percent of Caucasian North Americans, 40 percent of African North Americans and Hispanics and nearly 70 percent of Japanese North Americans (who, as it happens, have a very high rate of stomach cancer).

You can use food to tweak Phase I and Phase II enzymes: garlic, milk thistle, green tea and full-spectrum grape extract all slow down levels of Phase I enzymes; broccoli contains indole-3-carbinol, calcium D-glutarate and alpha lipoic acid that boost levels of Phase II enzymes; and the lignans from flax seeds also boost the efficiency of Phase II enzymes. Each day, use a large variety of colorful vegetables, sprouts, salad, fresh fruit, herbs and spices to help your detoxification process.

Raymond's Ultra Fast CT Scans Are Finding Out What My Grandma Knew

My grandmother began the first fresh, organic vegetable juice outlet in Hollywood, California nearly sixty years ago. She was a Hollywood legend and a health food pioneer before there were natural food stores. She earned the enduring nickname "Herbs, Nuts, Twigs and Seeds."

Nana Marie was a vegetarian, an herbalist, an environmentalist and a raw food advocate. Daily, she would make fresh vegetable juices with a minimal amount of carrots, but concentrated mostly on rich sources of chlorophyll and live enzymes. She used watercress, parsley, kale, Swiss chard, cilantro, red beets, a tomato, mustard greens, wheat grass and both radish and broccoli sprouts. She would include herbs like milk thistle and spices like garlic, turmeric, cloves, ginger and at times, cinnamon.

As an herbalist and natural food advocate, she knew that cruciferous vegetables, sprouts, bitter vegetables, herbs and spices protected the human body against the genotoxicity caused by both dietary and environmental carcinogens. She would affectionately say, "Have a glass of fresh juice packed with chlorophyll, a pure green-gold elixir." She would generally continue, "Honey boy, this is pure nectar of the gods, your guaranteed antidote to all this pollution."

Nana Marie intuitively knew that each of these potent, cell-friendly foods would love us back by preferentially detoxifying and inhibiting specific exotoxin environmental compounds from initiating a cancerous reaction. They could simply disarm and eliminate exotoxin chemicals called xenobiotics, and spark both a strong immune response and Phase I and Phase II elimination pathways.

Jane Fonda, Barbra Streisand and so many other Hollywood personalities would come to Nana Marie daily for her legendary organic juices spiked with beneficial, natural compounds, now linked to protection against cancer and cardiovascular disease. It was a remarkable sight to see. Mid-afternoon she would ask me to pray with her, specifically for all the suffering people in the world, then enter into quiet meditation.

Cutting-Edge Research: Catching Up with Grandma

Today, high-tech researchers like Raymond Rodriguez are clinically proving what my grandmother already knew. Daily, you can use cell-friendly foods, sprouts, herbs and spices to effectively tweak and boost Phase I and Phase II enzyme reactions to quickly initiate biotransformation of environmental exotoxins (xenobiotics) before they can injure your 100 trillion delicately crafted and most faithful cells. This is your way to love your cells right back!

I'm betting on Nana Marie, because I believe microbiologists shortly will also discover that parsley, kale, Swiss chard, mustard, red beets, tomatoes, cilantro, all sprouts, all herbs, cloves, ginger, garlic, turmeric and cinnamon will prove to be nature's powerful bi-functional inducers of both Phase I and Phase II metabolic detoxifying enzymes.

Nana Marie would probably say, "Those lab researchers need a good glass of vegetable juice to know exactly what it can do." Job well done, Nana Marie. Yes, Nana Marie was a Wise Elder, probably just like your grandmother and grandfather!

Assessing Phase I and Phase II Efficiency

To assess Phase I and Phase II efficiency, a patient takes three mild toxins: caffeine, acetaminophen (Tylenol) and aspirin. Since caffeine is almost completely metabolized by Phase I reactions, a saliva sample taken a few hours after the caffeine ingestion will indicate how well the Phase I pathway works. Acetaminophen and aspirin require both Phase I and Phase II for their elimination. By doing a simple analysis of blood and urine the following morning, the ability of the liver to detoxify environmental chemicals, toxins and carcinogens can be accurately assessed.

Candida Albicans (Yeast) Overgrowth

An overgrowth of "bad bugs" such as harmful yeast and other pathogenic organisms causes an imbalance in normal intestinal bacteria and is called *dysbiosis*. Dysbiosis can affect up to 60 percent of women and causes PMS, headaches, chronic fatigue syndrome and depression. The most commonly prescribed medication for dysbiosis, most commonly experienced as a yeast overgrowth, candida micro-organism infestation, is Diflucan (fluconazole) at $10 a day and with side effects including nausea, vomiting and diarrhea. Nystatin (Mucostatin) is prescribed in less serious cases of yeast overgrowth and costs $1 a day, with virtually no side effects.

The natural anti-yeast plan prescribed by the progressive and dedicated women's specialist Carolyn DeMarco, MD, is to eliminate sugar, "yeasty" foods (cheeses, vinegar, mushrooms, wine, breads, beer), and processed foods from your diet, and supplement with probiotics such as acidophilus and bifidus "friendly" bacteria, along with "green foods" rich in chlorophyll, caprylic acid, olive leaf extract, grapefruit seed extract, garlic capsules, oregano oil, aloe vera juice, and a daily detox formula to rid the colon of dead yeast from the "die-off" reaction that could otherwise make you feel worse than you felt before.

Exploring Your Inner Space

There is a small instrument being used for medical diagnosis of the digestion and absorption functions. Called the M2A gut cam, the pill-sized device developed by Given Imaging Ltd. allows doctors to take a trip through your GI tract. After being swallowed, the capsule takes fifty-seven thousand images of its voyage before being expelled and retrieved. The device's movements are recorded in real time by eight sensors placed on your abdomen.

Dr. Aleksandar Radan, a critical care medicine and surgery specialist, told me, "These vessels are a new class of small, potentially disposable, wireless technologies. The technologies for making these miniature devices are becoming more accessible." Interestingly, implantable diagnostic devices are rapidly shrinking, and there are already blood-cell-size nanobot monitoring devices on the drawing boards of half-a-dozen high-tech companies.

By the year 2015, medical researchers predict that nanobots will be removing toxins, xenobiotics, pathogens and intracellular trash from your cells, while repairing any damage this garbage may have caused to your tissues. However, "Today it is critically important that you make all the wise lifestyle choices to reduce your exposure to environmental carcinogens and toxins while optimizing your body's Phase I and Phase II detoxification capabilities," states Dr. Radan.

TURN DOWN THE HEAT AND IMPROVE THE DETOX PROCESS WITH INFRARED SAUNAS

There are new infrared saunas you can now install in your home or use at a health clinic. The infrared thermal heat penetrates three times deeper than regular saunas. Infrared heaters heat the skin and deeper tissues to three inches, cleansing deep tissues effectively. You also sweat twice as much as regular saunas in cooler, more tolerable temperatures of 110 to 130 degrees Fahrenheit. Measurable amounts of metabolic waste, such as PCBs, hydrocarbons and amphetamine metabolites are cleansed from the body rather than silently accumulating and growing. I use an infrared heated sauna several times a week; see the Product Reference section at the back of the book for a supplier. Be sure to drink lots of water while in a sauna.

13

SPIRITUAL INSIGHTS: BE INSPIRED

THE LAUGHTER OF LIFE

Happiness and Laughter: Cell-Friendly Mood Menders

Sometimes you may find yourself looking in the mirror and wondering if it's really possible to regain some of your youthful vitality and dynamic wellness. You're at an important crossroads and you can go either way. Many of your family or friends have given up, but you do not have to. All that's required is knowledge, encouragement and inspiration. Are you willing to work for it?

Happiness is a pure stress buster that is as helpful as body-ready nutrition and fitness. Laughter is contagious, supportive and beneficial for yourself and everyone around you. How many times have you seen humor diffuse a tense situation, ease some pain or open a door to deeper understanding? Laughter and good humor are soothing signals that ripple through the individual and all of society because they help to lift us all to joy.

Laughter Is Good Exercise

What else can so enjoyably exercise the heart and boost your mood? Laughter can serve as a social signal and a good mood lubricant. It enhances happiness and lightheartedness. The physical and psychological benefits of laughter are the subject of serious scientific study.

Laughter may not only create a wordless bond, it may well protect us from disease. Doctors tell patients to exercise to help heart function and respiration rate, boost moods, oxygenate the tissues, reduce levels of the stress hormone cortisol and, most importantly, reduce the likelihood of repeated heart attacks. Robert Provine, psychologist and neuroscientist at the University of Maryland, author of *Laughter: A Scientific Investigation*, realizes from his research that laughing accomplishes these very same mind-body benefits. Surprisingly, laughter makes your body alkaline.

The Healing Power of Laughter

Laughter is the best medicine for mind and body. Scientific studies have shown that laughter can strengthen the immune system, raise pain thresholds and ease depression. We all need to be encouraged to lighten up and open up to the wonder and delight of life.

Research conducted at the Department of Behavioral Medicine at the UCLA Medical School into the physical benefits of laughter proved conclusively that "laughter, happiness and joy are perfect antidotes for stress." Psychiatrist Dr. Abram Hoffer said that "the diaphragm, thorax, abdomen, heart, lungs—even the liver—are given a highly beneficial massage during a hearty laugh."

Crystal Andrus, author of the highly acclaimed *Simply...Woman*! says, "In the near future a doctor's recommendation for a healthy heart, for more energy or to relieve depression may one day be eat healthy food, exercise, sleep soundly and laugh deeply a few times a day."

Creation is a marvelous divine play that assigns each of us a different role. Not taking life or yourself too seriously does not mean being irresponsible. In actuality, you become more responsible by being aware of the magic and mystery in every moment. Laughter is the nectar of present moment awareness. Laughter is a quality of spirituality. Laughter is the tingling flow of love, coursing through your 100 trillion cells.

One of my favorite poets is the 14th century Persian mystic Hafiz, who writes:

What is laughter?
What is this precious love and laughter
Budding in our hearts?
It is the glorious sound
Of a soul waking up!

Using Laughter as Mind-Body Medicine

Laughter clubs are here. Borrowing an idea from Indian physician and famed laughing doctor Madan Kataria, psychologist Steve Wilson has launched a therapeutic-laughter group at website www.worldlaughtertour.com or www.jesthealth.com, offering training for what he calls Certified Laughter Leaders. The Laughter Leaders establish clubs in schools, prisons, half-way homes, hospitals, nursing homes and substance abuse rehabilitation centers to bond people together, getting them laughing and feeling a whole lot happier. Laughing is a way to blow off steam and discharge internal tension.

The Laughter Infection

Dr. Kataria, forty-six in 2005, started his first laughing group in 1998. His formula for getting people to laugh proved infectious. There are eighteen hundred such clubs in India alone, and an additional eight hundred around the world from Finland to Japan. Wendy, thirty-eight in 2005 and a police officer, told me, "There is a lot of pressure in my job, but now when I get stressed, anxious, annoyed or emotionally overwhelmed, I just have a good hearty laugh and it is gone."

What if you don't feel like laughing? No problem with faking it: Your brain and body don't know the difference. Dr. Kataria says, "Laughter can't solve your irritability, tension, stress, raging or problems, but it can quickly dissolve them." Brain scans prove that laughter can help lower blood pressure and cholesterol levels, raise chances of survival after a heart attack, reduce loneliness, depression and foul moods and quickly send all-round good cheer throughout your brain, body, heart and soul—and way beyond!

Lightheartedness

Play and laughter go hand in hand. Play is an opportunity to recreate yourself. When you are playing you lose track of time. This timeless domain, touched in play, is the realm of spirit. Spirit is pure creative force and spirit is innately playful.

You are a human being, capable of exploring your own origins. Now you have the opportunity and capacity to experience the exquisite combination of mature wisdom and a revitalized mind-body-mood-spirit connection.

THE BREATH OF LIFE

The Miracle of Cell-Friendly Oxygen

Optimal health and spiritual wellness are impossible without optimal breathing. This may seem self-evident, but most people breathe shallowly—just enough to get by.

It is a revelation to suddenly recharge with oxygen and watch your energy soar.

Restoring the healthy integration between your mind, body, mood and spirit by using conscientious breathing techniques brings about a renewal. To give yourself a natural energy boost and to keep yourself relaxed and clearheaded, stay conscious of your breathing. Breathe fully, completely and deeply. Avoid places that have poor or stagnant air, such as smoke-filled rooms.

We are alive because green vegetation makes the oxygen we need to live and uses our exhaled toxic carbon dioxide as food. Oxygen is the most important cell-friendly nutrient of all. You can live thirty days without food and four days without water, but you die in four minutes without oxygen. People assume that they get all the oxygen they need by breathing, but your oxygen supply is determined by first, the depth of your breathing, and second, the quality of air you breathe.

The vital energy in the air we breathe is called *chi* by the Chinese, *ki* by the Japanese, and *prana* by those from India. Unfortunately, in North America we really don't have a name for it.

Only by Breathing Can You Recharge with Fresh Oxygen

You can also breathe unobtrusively during moments of anxiety or stress. It is an excellent natural relaxant and energy booster, helping you feel more in tune and connected physically, mentally, emotionally and spiritually. Practice slow, deep breathing while standing, sitting or lying down for as long as you like—one of life's greatest revitalizers. Your euphoria goes up a few notches when you recharge your cells with refreshing oxygen and get the toxins out. Daily, intentional, slow, deep breathing produces a natural oxygen high, bringing energy and exhilaration. Your mind and body quickly become in sync, your alertness soars and you feel more vibrant.

Practicing deep breathing will immediately balance your nervous system and heart rhythm, oxygenating the hemoglobin in your blood as it moves into the deep tissues of your heart, brain, organs, glands and intestines—in every one of your 100 trillion cells. Deep breathing makes your body oxygen rich (aerobic) and alkaline.

HOW TO BREATHE WITH RHYTHM

No one teaches us how to breathe well for optimum well-being. It is a shame. Right now, let your inhalation become a little deeper and your exhalation a little longer with each breath. Take several natural and effortless slow breaths like this and notice how you feel in sync.

Use your breath to de-stress personal rage, pain, disappointment, anger, embarrassment and irritability in your life and reduce the misery and pain in the world. Slowly inhale your pain, rage, anger or anxiety—then exhale and release a reconciled, cleansed, ventilated, calm emotional version. Then consider all the people in the world in your same situation or worse. Inhale global pain, prejudice, anger, frustration, violence, injustice and misery, then exhale transformed emotions that reduce global misery, pain and fear.

Breathing with attention and intention establishes a state of unity in which the body, mind and spirit are experienced as one continuum. This then allows you to carry out your daily activities without losing that magical connection to your *wholeness*. This is the ultimate goal of all techniques and practices designed to integrate your body-mind-mood-spirit. Breath imparts to you a force that is as measurable as an electromagnetic field. Trauma of any sort, or stress, can arrest your free breathing and, in turn, will often negatively affect your life-force. The unimpeded flow of oxygen—through both nostrils—is essential to balance every human being's life-force. Your breathing can be used to boost your spiritual awareness and help all humanity.

Simple Breathing Techniques for Greater Awareness

You can quickly energize and invigorate your body and mind with the breathing technique called "bellows breath." This breath increases oxygen flow to your cells and cleanses the lungs. More than an exchange of gases, the way we breathe has implications and consequences for our body, mind and spiritual planes.

Most of us use less than one-third of our lung capacity when we inhale and exhale.

Sit comfortably with a relaxed but straight back and close your eyes. Exhale all the air from your lungs. Then begin deep in-and-out breathing through your nose. Try to have a rhythm with your lungs acting like a "bellows." Use 2-second inhalations and 2-second exhalations. Do this for thirty repetitions.

Finally, end with five deep and slow inhalations and exhalations, about 10 seconds for each one. You will notice that your mind is clear, your body is full of lovely sensations and you feel energized and in sync. Never hyperventilate to the point of feeling light-headed or dizzy.

You can also use your breathing in self-guided imagery and visualizations to reduce stress from information overload, if you feel crunched time-wise, or you feel trapped. Imagery provides the right brain with non-verbal oblique messages of reassurance, peace of mind, and safety. It calms us with moderately compelling biofeedback images and multi-sensory ideas. It distracts the thinking brain from its obsessive list of worries.

Breathe slowly and close your eyes. Visualize your dilemma or acute stress and let it float away on a balloon or cloud; or take out a shoebox in your mind, put your dilemma or stress in the box and deal with it later. When you use imagination to reduce stress or anxiety, you learn ways to avoid "thinking traps."

> Stop the words now.
> Open the windows in the center of your chest,
> and let Spirit fly in and out.
> Rumi, 12th century Persian mystic poet

THE CREATIVITY OF LIFE

Convergent thinking aims for a single, correct solution to a problem by using logic to find an orthodox solution and to determine if it is unambiguously right or wrong. IQ tests primarily involve convergent thinking. But creative people can free themselves from conventional thought patterns to follow new neural pathways to unique or distantly associated answers. This ability is known as divergent thinking, which can generate many unique, possible answers. Creativity is divergent thinking in action.

Steps to Enhance Your Creativity and Divergent Thinking

Courage. Strive to think outside accepted principles and habitual perspectives.

Motivation. As soon as a spark of genuine interest arises in something, follow up.

Relaxation. Take the time to daydream and ponder; that is often when the best ideas arise.

Wonderment. Try to retain a spirit of discovery and a child-like curiosity.

"If prayer is like talking to God, meditation is a way of listening to the divine within."

Edgar Cayce

THE MEDITATION OF LIFE

While most people have become familiar with meditation through eastern religions, Christianity, Islam and Judaism have powerful and ancient meditation practices as well. In fact, all the world's religions have meditation traditions as the central devotional activity in their quest for connection with their belief of the Divine.

Our Brain and Neuroscience

We all have feelings of loneliness, inadequacy, self-doubt, fear, anxiety or the blues from time to time. Fortunately, they do not have to dominate our lives.

At Harvard's School of Public Health, University of Wisconsin, University of Alberta in Edmonton, UC Berkeley and Stanford University, researchers using two brain-imaging technologies—electroencephalographs (EEG), which sense the electrical activity of neuronal circuits, and functional magnetic resonance imaging (fMRI), which maps blood flow to active parts of the brain—consistently point to the left prefrontal cortex as the primary site of contentment, happiness, joy, feelings of deep connectedness, healthy self-esteem and a sense of unity and oneness. It is not a vague random state but one you can induce deliberately.

The brain rewires itself in response to new experiences, especially if the experience is practiced daily.

Only over the last decade, neuroscientists like Dr. Richard Restak, of George Washington University Medical Center in Washington, D.C., and many others have learned that the human brain is not static and stationary, but very fluid and pliable, constantly reshaping and renewing itself. Just as the structure and function of the heart changes—improving or deteriorating—in response to diet, stress, exercise and lifestyle, so do those of the brain.

The Current View of Consciousness—"*Now*"

Meditation is one such experience that allows us to not only bounce back from unpleasant emotions, but to actually rewire our brain for a revitalized look at ourselves and the miracle of our human experience in this universe. Science is proving that meditation strengthens our peaceful equanimity muscle and vaccinates against fear, depression, anxiety, insecurity and melancholy. Not surprisingly, for some this is an opportunity to go beyond sensory pleasures into the timeless, spaceless region of *now*!

"If the doors of perception were cleansed every thing would appear to man just as it is, infinite."

William Blake, artist and poet

A New View of Consciousness

The real essence of this book is to encourage you to tap into your inner reservoir and grasp greater wisdom, meaning, joy, compassion, faith and hope in your life. We are the most blessed and fortunate of any species because we can instantly change our perceptions, interpretations, limiting restrictions, and expectations of our life experience and open up to a new, unrestricted reality of ourselves.

Despite how radical some of these timeless, boundless experiences may appear at first, if you earnestly try them, you will be amazed at your results.

Meditation and Prayer

WHAT HAPPENS WHEN YOU MEDITATE: PART I

fMRIs prove that the left prefrontal cortex of the brain, a center of higher mental functioning, is enhanced in meditation or deep prayer. What does this mean? It means you can improve your brain's biological structure and electrochemical wiring all life long, while reducing stress and making yourself happy.

During meditation, when you enter the gap between thoughts, time stops. This was the basis of the psychological concept of flow. When we glimpse the realm of spirit through meditation, or an awe-inspiring experience, we enter a state of consciousness that is beyond time and space. There is a silent witness within, not restricted to any particular experience, or time, or place. It is the same presence that existed before we were born, when we were born, when we were children, teenagers, adults and *now*. This is the essence of who we are.

In meditation we want to quietly shift our attention to this *now*, the only non-changing state in a life of constant change. When our attention is on our physical well-being, our material possessions, our to-do list or our fears, our awareness is focused on the real but impermanent objective reality.

A shift in consciousness from object-oriented reality to our inner witness or Self is a shift from time-bound, place-bound awareness (mind-body interactions) to timeless and placeless awareness. Your Self is the only timeless, boundless, pure state in the midst of time-bound experiences of the objective world.

When we maintain this inner silence, inner peace, inner centeredness, even in the midst of an active, time-driven world, we will experience a new relationship with time and each of our life experiences.

Be A Witness—No Judgment or Critique

Another way to experience the timeless state of mind is to become aware of the pause between breaths, between our physical movements, between our thoughts. Then we go beyond the constant chatter of internal dialogue and enter the timeless state of *now*!

Deep, Slow Breathing

Yet another way to experience the timeless state of mind is to become aware of our breath without controlling it. Do not forcefully exaggerate your breath. Simply follow it in and out. Inhale. Exhale. Relax into the timeless state of *now*!

Sincere Prayer

The most traditional and time-proven western way to experience the timeless state of mind is to enter into selfless prayer—dialogue with the

Divine. Spontaneous, free-flowing conversations allow our thoughts and background noise to dissipate, evaporate, leaving only the *now*. When Moses was at the top of Mount Sinai with the burning bush and he asked by what name the Divine could be called, the answer was "I am that I am." St. Paul talks about deep prayer and union as "The peace that surpasses all understanding," and the Psalms state "Be still and know that I am God"—the timeless state of *now*!

WHAT HAPPENS WHEN YOU MEDITATE: PART II

Our bodies look static in meditation or prayer, because the perception of *now* is too subtle to be directly perceived with the senses even though radical awarenesses are occurring. Consider our bodies. Every six months we replace the calcium in our bones. In just one month we replace all the cells in our skin. In about four months our heart has been reshaped and remodelled because every cell is renewed and reconstructed. Consider a babbling brook. At any one spot the brook may appear the same, but in actuality it, like our bodies, is simultaneously and continually changing and renewing, even if we are not consciously aware of it.

Even if we are not aware that at every moment all our cells, atoms and subatomic molecules are constantly changing, they are. The same holds true for the babbling brook. Nothing in this physical universe is static, stationary. Everything is constantly changing and renewing itself.

Each of us is a dynamic, conscious entity rather than fixed, stationary matter. Life is really a cosmic dance. We must be open to the inexhaustible and constant transformation of fluid consciousness. We must see our true essence not as limited, time-bound, restricted or static, but eternally in dynamic relationship with the universe. "Seek and ye shall find, knock and it shall be opened unto thee."

We can then experience and perceive even our bodies as subtle energy, not stationary matter. What is fascinating is that reliable EEGs in brain wave studies show improved interactions between different parts of the brain during meditation. For instance, your consumption of oxygen during meditation decreases by 50 percent—as much as during deep sleep. These changes are not seen during our wakeful times.

Even more revealing, your everyday waking brain waves, in order to be efficient and productive, are busy beta waves in the range of 13–39 cycles per second (13–39 Hz). In a deeply relaxed meditative state, your brain relaxes to a vibration that measures about 8 cycles per second (8 Hz). Amazingly, this field links up with the frequency of the earth's electromagnetic field. You are one with nature then, content, at home, connected and grounded. If you go into very deep meditation, prayer or "flow" you can experience gamma synchrony at 60 to 90 Hz, which is a reorganizing and binding of all sensory and cognitive functions of the brain for better brainpower and a deep sense of contentment. Your cellular machinery and DNA were not designed to deal with 900 MHz cell phone frequencies. Take steps to reduce electromagnetic exposure while using your cell phone by attaching magnetic ferrite beads to it.

A NEW FERTILITY FACTOR

Anne was thirty-three when I first met her and her husband, Steve. She had been trying to get pregnant for more than five years. All she gained after several cycles of injected fertility medication were 10 extra pounds. I encouraged her to give up alcohol and caffeine, to eat only cell-friendly foods, to start practicing relaxation techniques and to begin to meditate for half-an-hour with Steve each morning and evening. After three months she conceived. Her son arrived nine happy months later. Though practices like meditation certainly can't guarantee pregnancy, it has now established its effectiveness along with high-tech medicines and procedures.

RELAXING FRAZZLED NERVES

When emotional stress disrupts mind-body communication, the effects can be seen on a brain scan. An area known as the midcingulate cortex goes into accelerated overdrive. Stress-related digestive problems, as well as sleep-related problems, have potentially devastating consequences.

Dave, thirty-five, came to me as a stressed-out, recovering alcoholic and recreational drug user. I told Dave that meditation, stress reduction, deep breathing and cell-friendly foods were an effective alternative to an antidepressant he was advised to use. His doctor agreed.

Meditation helped Dave quell the amplification of stress by reorienting destructive ways of thinking. Meditation calmed his exaggerated heart and nervous systems and tuned down red-alert signals from cortisol and adrenaline, replacing them with calming but alert serotonin and DHEA. In four weeks Dave noticeably improved and over time recovered, becoming the father of two lovely children and a counselor for drug abusers in prison. Dave learned to identify the early signs of an emotional hurricane—fatigue, irritability, frustration—before it hits. "I am at peace now," he says, because he knows what affects his emotional trigger points and how to de-stress.

Meaningful Pauses

You do not need a self-help manual; you only have to meditate. Another form of meditation is called "meaningful pauses," which can literally create a healing response to any acute stress, illness, pain or suffering. "Meaningful pauses" are short, 3-minute, mindful periods throughout the day of quiet, deep breathing to reduce pain and anxiety.

HAVING A HEALTHY, HAPPY HEART

At every stage of heart disease, state of mind appears to play a role. "Diet and exercise alone are like a two-legged stool," says Dr. Redford Williams, director of the Behavioral Medicine Research Center at Duke University. "It is more stable with the third leg—effective stress management." Dr. Dean Ornish states, "Patients in our studies showed a 91 percent reduction in angina, with diet and stress reduction, in a few weeks to a few months without the trauma or expense of angioplasty or bypass surgery." Genetic profiling is the newest technology used to pinpoint who could benefit the most by any particular intervention. A Dutch study of elderly heart patients showed that daily stress-reduction periods reduced an individual's risk of death by 50 percent over the study's nine-year duration.

Maria had suffered the agony of arthritic joint pain in her fingers and spine. Painkillers dulled the aches, but relief didn't come until she discovered a powerful pain-reduction medication inside her own body: her mind. She uses "meaningful pauses" every hour. It is intended to become a way of life.

SOOTHING A SENSITIVE GUT

It has probably happened to you. You're driving to work or school and suddenly remember that a neglected assignment is due today. Your stomach clenches, your intestines twist and shiver, and before you know it, you feel sick. Research points out that one in four people end up seeking medical attention for a gastrointestinal problem such as indigestion, irritable bowel syndrome (IBS) or heartburn. Doctors test for ulcers or tumors and find that everything is normal—but it is not!

When emotional distress disrupts the dialogue along the mind-body communication network of neurotransmitters (in this case, from the stomach to the brain), hormones and peptides, the effects can be seen on a brain scan. The scan shows that you suffer devastating consequences because an area in the brain known as the midcingulate cortex goes into an immediate overdrive. Mind-body techniques like deep breathing, progressive relaxation, biofeedback, soothing exercises like Tai Chi or hatha yoga, and meditation can provide a safe, effective alternative to antacids and anti-diarrhea medications. These mind-body techniques can calm the autonomic nervous system and switch from the red-alert stress sympathetic dominance to the de-stressing, relaxed parasympathetic nervous system.

Don't Run Away from Conflict— Breathe It In and Out—Give It Fresh Air

Another form of meditation is conscientious breathing, taking in cleansing and purifying air and neutralizing destructive conflicts within ourselves or on behalf of others.

We must not run away from what we are afraid of: distasteful conflicts, embarrassing situations or personality clashes. Though they are points of rage, conflict, aggression and revenge for most people, they are also indicators of issues that we need to work on. Breathe in your rage, anger, disgust, embarrassment or conflict—without judgment—and breathe back out a fresh, relaxed exhalation, visualizing that you have cleansed and ventilated the "internal poison" and given it back to the world as a recycled, purified version. Do this for four or five breaths. Then realize that there are people in the world suffering the very same conflict or ailment as yourself at this very moment. Take their pain, suffering, anguish, despair, rage, hatred, injustice, revenge, prejudice, embarrassment, aggression and breathe it in for them. Breathe out a cleansed, reconciled, freshened emotional forgiveness for them and a healing for their spirits, hearts, nerves, mind, emotions and body. You are now concerned with global wellness and global healing as much as personal wellness and personal healing.

This mindful approach regards what happens in our lives as useful lessons, and realizes that the path itself is not to be avoided.

Be Realistic, Be Loving and Be Part of the Solution

Joy, as events remind us, is a fragile state. In the sufferings of millions in the Asian tsunami or in the anguish of war, in the sorrow of bereavement, in the grief following 9/11, in the bewilderment of forest fires and avalanches, and in the horror of earthquakes and the devastation of floods, it has become clearer than ever how all of life's tremors—personal, economic, political and tectonic—can sometimes make the pursuit of happiness seem trivial, yet we cannot live without joy and happiness.

A PRIMARY MEDITATION TECHNIQUE

- Sit in a quiet place and adopt a comfortable posture with your spine straight. If you are sitting cross-legged on the floor, you may find it helpful to straighten your spine by tucking a firm cushion under your pelvis. You may also sit in a straight-back chair.
- Let go of any tension in your body.
- Become aware of your breath and start slow breathing.
- Now let your breathing find its own rhythm. Bring your awareness to the place in your body where your breath arises. With each exhalation, bring your awareness to the place that your breath goes.
- Whenever your mind wanders, bring it back to the breath. There is no need to resist your thoughts as such—simply become aware that your focus has shifted to your thoughts and gently bring it back to the breath.
- Once you feel the quiet, equanimity and tranquility, ask for guidance and direction in your life. Ask that peace, love, compassion

and gratitude grow richly in your life. Breathe in any conflicts in your mind and breathe out a resolved, fresh version.
- Stay calm and undisturbed. Gently and attentively, with no effort, listen.
- Allow gratitude and blessedness to flow through the core of your being. If you are not flooded with gratitude and blessedness, you may not be meditating but still trying to force your will. *Let it go. Let it be.* Inhale the control, let go, and exhale the control.

Do this meditation exercise for at least 20 minutes daily, ideally at the beginning and/or end of the day. This is as rejuvenating as a 1-hour power nap.

At the very least, meditation or sincere prayer will dissolve and move you beyond self-limiting negative patterns. I think that every one of your 100 trillion cells would simply love that, and love you right back.

Spiritual Fitness Supplements

The ten main supplements to foster spiritual fitness are:

1. Inspirational and/or holy reading for an emotional transfusion
2. Daily mindfulness, including humanitarian efforts, which are mood menders
3. Writing spiritual poems, stories or letters (sent or unsent)
4. Reflective grace or thanksgiving before all meals or snacks (food and nourishment, as a real art, merge science and spirituality)
5. The magnificent spiritual power of inspiration: music, drumming, dancing, singing, laughing, forgiveness, kindness and compassion
6. Meditation, prayer or deep reflection at day's end
7. Spiritual guidance from a minister, priest, rabbi, Wise Elder, grandparent, trusted friend, or trained psychologist
8. Calm, deep breathing to de-stress and calm a tense body, anxious mind, agitated emotions or depressed moods; foster global well-being; and make your body alkaline
9. Positive affirmations from you to yourself, a miracle method to heal inner pain

10. Truthfulness about how you feel. Cry or release unexpressed restrictive emotions to liberate your subconscious feelings, and you will probably find yourself feeling lighter, happier, maybe even elated. Your owner's manual should come with one simple instruction—release once and for all any restrictive, limiting emotions.

    Become a Wise Elder for your own sake, and for global well-being.

"What you hold, may you always hold! What you do, may you always do and never abandon. But with swift pace, light step, unswerving feet, so that even your steps stir up no dust—may you go forward securely, joyfully and swiftly, on the path of prudent awakening."

Saint Clare of Assisi

Part IV

REJUVENATE

14

TWENTY-ONE WAYS TO TWEAK YOUR LIFESTYLE

When it comes to healthy habits, you now have most of your bases covered: you eat lots of colorful fruits and vegetables, take the stairs instead of the elevator, wisely supplement, exercise, practice deep breathing, get deep sleep and now you're meditating.

But no matter how impeccable you think your routine is, there are always ways to take it to the next level. All it takes is a few fast, easy refinements. These twenty-one simple lifestyle adjustments will bring out the healthiest, happiest you.

1 **Healthy Habit:** You like to drink herbal teas for wellness. **Kick It Up:** Both green and black teas come from the leaves of the plant *Camellia sinensis*. Green tea, however, undergoes less processing than black tea, thus preserving more of the protective phytonutrients called polyphenols, known cancer cell suppressors. The benefits of green tea are dose-dependent, in other words, the more green tea you drink, the greater the amount of epigallocatechin gallate (EGCG), the strongest anticancer polyphenol in green tea. Each morning, put four bags of organic green tea in a thermos with 4 cups of boiling water and 1 tablespoon of freshly chopped ginger and let it steep for 1 hour. It takes 1 hour for the EGCG to diffuse into the water. Drink this invigorating, anti-carcinogenic beverage throughout the day.

2 **Healthy Habit:** You like to spend time in peace and quiet daily.
Kick It Up: Listen to inspiring music or a meditative tape that will lift you from the noisy, bustling world and return you to a calming but alert alpha state and enhanced gamma synchrony. Listen to it while going to or from work, at lunch or before sleep to calm frazzled nerves. The wonderful CD of meditative songs that I like is *Daybreak in My Soul* by Elvira Clare. Search www.theforestofpeace.com to hear clips from the CD and to access further information.

3 **Healthy Habit:** You like color and fresh flowers.
Kick It Up: Every Monday morning bring a bouquet of brilliantly colored flowers to work—red, yellow, green and purple are great energizing colors. "You actually have a psychological response to colors that makes you feel revitalized," writes Leatrice Eiseman, author of *Colors For Every Mood.*

4 **Healthy Habit:** You eat salad.
Kick It Up: Trade iceberg lettuce for darker greens like spinach, coriander, parsley, watercress and mesclun. Dark greens are packed with vitamin A, folic acid, vitamin B9, alpha and beta carotene, and lutein, an antioxidant that can help prevent free radical damage that can cause cataracts. Also add daikon, radish, garlic, broccoli, and sunflower sprouts.

5 **Healthy Habit:** You brush your teeth regularly.
Kick It Up: Your toothbrush is a haven for germs to grow on. Before you use your toothbrush and immediately after, to kill the many hitch-hiking germs on it, put ten drops of hydrogen peroxide on your toothbrush, leave it for 5 seconds and rinse it off.

6 **Healthy Habit:** You volunteer once or twice a year.
Kick It Up: Commit yourself to volunteer on a regular basis, perhaps one weekend a month. Studies show that volunteering releases the "tend and befriend" hormone oxytocin and the "feel good" neuropeptide beta endorphins, increases both self-esteem and social-esteem, and relieves stress.

7 **Healthy Habit:** To sleep deeply, you watch what you eat after supper.

Kick It Up: Set your bedroom temperature at a lower level, around 65 degrees Fahrenheit, or 16 degrees Celsius. From my previous book, *The Food Connection*: "This is best for sleeping, since your body is not trying to adjust to being too hot or too cold."

8 **Healthy Habit:** You limit salt, sugar and saturated fats.

Kick It Up: Enjoy the experience of eating for its own sake, and savor the textures and flavors of your meals. This will allow you to have a healthy relationship with food and not become obsessed with counting numbers on labels. Say a grace or thanksgiving before eating. Always sit down to eat, and thoroughly chew and savor your cell-friendly food.

9 **Healthy Habit:** You like to wake up to coffee.

Kick It Up: Many studies indicate that up to 300 mg of caffeine a day, equal to the caffeine in about 2 cups of freshly brewed coffee, is safe. On a typical day, 70 percent of North American adults drink an average of 3.3 cups of coffee. Caffeine is effective only up to your "jitter threshold"; add more caffeine after this and you're too buzzed to think clearly. Research suggests that caffeine and its related methylxanthines enhance the release of two amino acids, glutamate and aspartate, which are the main excitatory neurotransmitters in the brain. The caffeine in coffee or tea can give you a mental alertness advantage if you are not caffeine-sensitive—that is, if you do not experience headaches, anxiety, jitters or irritability, and do not overdose on just half a cup of regular brewed coffee.

The *Journal of the National Cancer Institute* (on February 16, 2005) published research that suggests 85 percent of North Americans consume caffeine daily. Two studies established that coffee was linked to a decrease in liver cancer, and drinking coffee or tea was not associated with the risk of colon cancer.

If you do use caffeine in coffee or tea, limit your use to 2 cups a day, before noon. Coffee is one of the most heavily sprayed crops. Use organic coffee or tea to avoid exposure to toxic herbicides, pesticides and fertilizers. If you drink decaffeinated coffee, look for the "Swiss Water Process" method, which does not use chemicals to decaffeinate the coffee. If you use a drip coffeemaker, use unbleached filters. The bright white ones, which most people use, are chlorine bleached and some of this chlorine will be extracted from the filter during the brewing process. Only use certified, free trade, organic coffee or tea displaying a free trade logo, the most common ones being Fairtrade Labelling Organization International (FLO) and fair trade certified (FTC).

Dr. Charles Czeisler, a neuroscientist and sleep expert at Harvard Medical School, warns that "We use caffeine to make up for a sleep deficit that is largely the result of using caffeine." The new consensus view of coffee by most researchers is that caffeine is not dangerous at moderate levels of consumption—up to 300 mg or two 12-ounce cups of coffee a day. Repeated studies have shown that caffeine is analeptic (it stimulates the central nervous system) and ergogenic (it improves physical performance). It is also a diuretic, increasing urine output, but only about the same as water. Caffeine boosts blood pressure, too, but this effect is temporary. Some studies have shown that caffeine increases a tiny amount of calcium loss, so small that it could be replaced with as little as two tablespoons of milk a day. The best scientifically written book on the pros and cons of caffeine use is outlined in *The Caffeine Advantage* by Bennett A. Wernberg and Bonnie K. Bealie.

Parents should be aware of caffeinated soft drinks and iced tea. Besides the stimulative effects, an additional concern is that "pop" is acidifying and contains either a high sugar or synthetic sweetener content. We don't assume that children have the judgment to regulate their own consumption of such substances. An 8 oz cup of Arabica coffee contains an average of 150 mg of caffeine; 8 oz of green tea has 10–15 mg; and some soft drinks average 55 mg per 12 oz drink.

The Kola Nut—A Better Alternative to Coffee

We have created a kind of guilt by association with coffee, or specifically caffeine, that is not scientifically based. I have spent two years vigorously researching caffeine. I have discovered that the seeds of the kola nut (*Cola nitida*), a plant of the cacao plant family, are 3 percent caffeine and do not tax the adrenal glands like high-dose caffeine does. If you consume 80 to 160 mg of naturally occurring caffeine from the kola nut daily, it will give you an energetic boost, enhanced mental performance, and an ergogenic drive, but will not overstimulate your central nervous system. When combined with the amino acids taurine, tyrosine and glycine; vitamins B6 and C; traditional adaptogenic herbs like rhodiola rosea; and the trace mineral chromium, naturally occurring caffeine further enhances your supercritical energy while balancing your moods without the morning jitters or afternoon black clouds associated with drinking excessive coffee. This scientific combination of food-based nutrients and fiber balances your adrenal glands, blood sugar levels and critical insulin levels—while a sweetened coffee will raise them. Remember, Dr. Robert Dickson of Georgetown University explains that a powerful antioxidant found in the cacao plants called pentamer is a potent anticancer compound that causes apoptosis (death) of cancer cells.

10 **Healthy Habit:** On your days off you want to recharge.

Kick It Up: Get as far away from your work, mentally and physically, as you can—and keep busy, suggests Alice D. Domar, PhD, director of the Mind-Body Center for Women's Health in Boston. Sitting around unoccupied lets your mind drift to work topics, and the next thing you know, you're stressed out, thinking of all the things you will have to do when you go back. Get outside for a hike, go swimming, take a sauna, go to an exercise class or tackle home projects.

11 **Healthy Habit:** You take warm baths to wind down.

Kick It Up: Seek out water all day long: jog in light rain or eat lunch by a waterfall. Studies show that water, particularly falling water, has a significant body-calming effect, says Norman Rosenthal, MD, a clinical professor of psychiatry at Georgetown University and author of *The Emotional Revolution*. Flowing water gives off chemical particles that may help you relax, and the sound of falling water can soothe your nerves and gladden your heart.

12 **Healthy Habit**: You keep a positive attitude even during bad times, such as a relationship break-up or a stressful situation at work or home.

Kick It Up: Actively seek out happiness by looking for small moments of joy every day. For example, get up early and stretch outside as you watch a gorgeous sunrise. "Appreciating the little things can help you feel happier and more content on a daily basis," explains Professor Emeritus Dr. A.V. Rao, Faculty of Medicine, University of Toronto.

13 **Healthy Habit:** When stress strikes, you take a few deep breaths to calm down.

Kick It Up: Take regular deep-breathing breaks—meaningful pauses—during the day to stop tension from forming in the first place. Try this quick and effective exercise from meditation instructor Tony Murdock's CD, *Toward Health and Wellness* (see www.towardstillness.com): Inhale through your nose, then exhale slowly through your mouth so your breath sounds like a long sigh rather than a rush of air. Repeat three or four times. Your blood pressure and stress hormone levels will decrease and you'll bring oxygen to your heart and brain, which promotes relaxation.

14 **Healthy Habit:** You have a supportive group of friends.

Kick It Up: Surround yourself with people who have the emotional balance and optimism you admire. "When you spend time with people who possess character traits you like, you make those traits a part of your own personality," explains Carolyn DeMarco, MD.

15 **Healthy Habit:** You get some outdoor time a few days a week.

Kick It Up: Get outside for at least 30 minutes every day, especially when the sun is shining. Routine exposure to sunlight wards off seasonal depression, particularly in the winter months, says Dr. Aslam Khan. A mere 10- to 15-minute daily dose stimulates your system to produce adequate amounts of vitamin D, which is crucial for bone health and to prevent cancer and depression. "The fresh air also helps you feel calmer and more alert," says Dr. Khan of Optima Health Solutions International, Vancouver, British Columbia. You can visit his organization's website at www.optimahealthsolutions.com.

16 **Healthy Habit**: You like to resolve negative experiences.

Kick It Up: Don't just forget—actively forgive by saying you're sorry and asking the other person to apologize as well. Hearing a genuine "I'm sorry" has an immediate positive physiological effect, lowering heart rate and blood pressure and reducing facial tension, according to a new study. "Researchers have also found that people who forgive themselves and others feel much more positive about life," states Louise L. Hay, author of *Everyday Positive Thinking*. Visit her website at www.hayhouse.com.

17 **Healthy Habit**: You regularly exercise and work out.

Kick It Up: "Swap your favorite workout. Doing the same thing over and over again can be de-energizing and boring. Without that extra effort your body does not make those feel good hormones called beta endorphins that boost your mood and overall sense of well-being. Runners can improve stamina by incorporating weight training; regular lifters may see new results by doing hatha yoga; cyclists could try skiing and skiers could try mountain bikes," states Dr. Laina Shulman, DC, Pure-Health Clinic, London, Ontario. For more information, email info@pure-health.com.

18 **Healthy Habit**: You avoid being down, bluesy or moody.

Kick It Up: Trivial everyday problems may, at times, seem unmanageable. You can suddenly feel tense and moody, and have a rapid heart beat, sweaty palms or pure anxiety.

To reduce physical or emotional stress and to resynchronize your adrenal glands, use the very progressive product that I use, called *the pure calm de-stress kit,* which contains therapeutic herbs that helps you deal with your stress and promotes a sense of calm safely and naturally. Sometimes called "Zen in a bottle," it increases formation of the inhibitory neurotransmitter gamma-aminobutyric acid (GABA), which chills you out quickly and soothes the nervous system.

It calms the sympathetic nervous system by tuning down overexaggerated levels of "excitatory" neurochemicals like red-alert adrenaline and corrosive cortisol. For more information, visit www.genuinehealth.com. Also, take a few deep breaths and smile or laugh to turn on your alkaline, parasympathetic nervous system. Research supports smiling and laughing for reducing depression, moodiness and irritability.

19

Healthy Habit: You eat cell-friendly foods to avoid illness.

Kick It Up: Eat foods that research has proven are potent cancer fighters.

Broccoli and broccoli sprouts turn on the GST enzyme and related genes.

- GST produces the body's master antioxidant, glutathione, which has anticancer effectiveness by blocking microtubules in out-of-sync breast, prostate and colon cancer cell colonies.
- Broccoli and broccoli sprouts contain sulforaphane and indole-3-carbinol, which boost Phase I and Phase II detoxification of intracellular carcinogens, metabolic waste and chemical intruders in the liver.

Turmeric turns off Cox-2 and 5-Lox inflammatory-producing enzymes.

- Curcumin, the yellow pigment in turmeric and an ingredient in curry, prevents heart disease, colon cancer, Alzheimer's disease and neurodegenerative disorders by turning off inflammation-causing Cox-2 and 5-Lox enzymes. India is the country that consumes the most turmeric (in curry) and has the lowest incidence of Alzheimer's disease in the world.

Deep green vegetables turn off Cox-2 enzymes and slow down HER-2 positive genes associated with breast cancer cell proliferation.

- Deep green vegetables contain chlorophyll and chlorophyllin, as well as a flavonoid, apigenin, that the Eppley Cancer Research Center found was a potent inhibitor of ultraviolet light-induced skin cancer and blocks the growth signals that skin cancer cells require to grow and spread. Chlorophyllin slows down HER-2 positive genes from sending growth signals to epidermal cancer cells and also turns off Cox-2 enzymes to reduce system-wide inflammation.

Garlic turns on the p53 gene.

- The p53 gene blocks the initiation or progression of colon, breast and prostate cancer cell colony formation, and signals cancer cells to self-destruct, a process called apoptosis.

Green tea slows down HER-2 positive genes.

- Green tea polyphenols, especially EGCG, turn off growth signals in breast, colon, prostate and skin cancer cells and demonstrate further anticancer effectiveness by protecting healthy cellular DNA structure. EGCG inhibits the metastasis of cancer cell colonies at the G2 stage. Somewhere between 20 to 30 percent of North American women genetically carry the HER-2 positive gene that appears to promote unusually rapid growth of breast tumors.

20

Healthy Habit: You want to avoid cravings and you also exercise to strengthen your heart and cardiovascular system.

Kick It Up: Exercise cures cravings for sweets. Interestingly, researchers have discovered a cure for sweet cravings and bingeing. Japanese investigators gave athletes the choice between two water bottles, one containing a sugar solution and the other containing just distilled water. The athletes had a tendency to drink more fluids if they liked the taste of the drink, particularly if the drink was sweet.

Amazingly, after exercising, the athletes' appetite for the sweet taste dramatically decreased. The researchers discovered that there is a dramatic reduction in insulin levels after exercise. Athletes preferred unsweetened water after exercise.

Elevated insulin levels are one of the primary reasons for food cravings, and if insulin levels are reduced, most of these cravings disappear.

So if you haven't already picked up the exercise habit—even brisk walking is sufficient—here is a powerful motivation to do so if you struggle with cravings for sweets. Eating sufficient protein at each of your three meals also reduces insulin levels by elevating the counter-regulatory, or antidote hormone, glucagon to balance exaggerated insulin surges. So exercise daily and never eat a meal without adequate protein, salad and vegetables. Note that when you eat anything sweet or starchy, your insulin levels increase. When insulin levels increase, you are sending a signal to your cells to store carbohydrates as fat and not to release any of the stored fat. This makes it impossible for you to burn and use up your own stored body fat for energy.

An Ancient Food to Prevent Heart Disease

Often compared to cheese because of its pungent aroma, natto consists of boiled soybeans that are fermented until they acquire their nutty flavor. Natto has been a traditional Japanese food for more than one thousand years. Ancient samurai consumed natto daily to increase their strength.

Natto is produced in a fermentation process by adding *Bacillus subtilis*, a beneficial bacteria, to boiled soybeans. The bacteria acts on the soybeans, producing the nattokinase enzyme, which has proven to be enormously successful for dissolving blood clots.

In 1928, Sir Alexander Fleming noted that a mold called *Penicillium notatum* stopped the growth of the staphylococci bacteria and, even more importantly, that it could be used in medicines to combat infectious diseases. Likewise, in 1980, Dr. Hiroyuki Sumi from the University of Chicago discovered nattokinase and its potent fibrinolytic (blood clot-busting) activity. The human body contains several enzymes, like fibrin, that promote the formation of blood clots, but it produces only one enzyme—plasminogen—that dissolves them. Nattokinase is very similar to plasminogen and is able to dissolve fibrin while enhancing the body's natural production of plasminogen. Eat natto several times a week or use one to three capsules daily between meals. Each capsule should contain at least 50 mg of natto extract with 1,100 fibrin units per capsule.

21

Healthy Habit: You like to be vibrant and energetic.

Kick It Up: Determine to be vibrant and energetic your entire life.

Silken Laumann, Canada's well-known Olympic rower, won a silver medal at the Atlanta Olympics in 1996. In 1998 she was inducted into Canada's Sports Hall of Fame. Silken approached me after one of my lectures and said, "I wish I would have known everything you are talking about when I was a competitive Olympic rower."

Be determined now to break away from society's belief that aging is equated with physical and mental deterioration. My brother, Joe Graci, did at 68 years of age, and now at 77 he is an energy dynamo.

If you continue to learn daily from your own life experiences and are ready for progressive change, you can increase your physical, mental, emotional and spiritual capacity. The more you replace cell-damaging choices with cell-friendly choices, the more profound will be your physical, mental, emotional and spiritual benefits all life long. Just one change in your perspective about aging or your expectation of yourself at any age determines the outcome. Since your body is a hologram—this means that the whole is contained in each and every cell or part—whenever one cell or part or expectation changes, everything else changes.

You must use this principle to your advantage. If you want a physician to check your cholesterol, insulin, estrogen and testosterone levels, only a tiny bit of blood is collected from a pin prick in your arm. Science accepts that what is true for that one drop of blood is true throughout your entire body. Use this principle to influence your entire well-being, energy and mood by simply making a positive healthy shift in your future expectations of your well-being. As you think, so you are—and so you will be.

If you expect your mental and physical capacity to decline with age, it will. If you change your expectation to the idea that growing older means growing better, with more knowledge, deeper spirituality, equanimity, peace, vitality, clarity and personal presence, this will be your experience.

WISE ELDER OR RAPIDLY AGING SENIOR

Vibrant seniors in many traditions are revered for their knowledge, depth, insight, spirituality and dynamic living presence. We call them Wise Elders.

I wholeheartedly ask that you seriously consider doing one of these lifestyle refinements each day for twenty-one days to coincide with your twenty-one-day diet adjustment so you can grow from ordinary to remarkable. Why stop short of your full potential?

Dr. Ellen Langer, a Harvard psychologist, performed an interesting study to highlight what I am recommending. She took groups of men in their seventies and eighties and encouraged them to think, act, talk and behave as if they were twenty-five years younger. After only seven days, the minimum time for change to begin to work, a number of physical traits associated with aging began to improve. Their hearing and vision sharpened, they had better joint mobility and they performed better on tests of manual dexterity. Their energy levels and good mood increased significantly. Your perceptions and expectations can determine the actual outcome—a self-fulfilling prophecy. Remember: as you think, so you are—and so you will be.

Become a Wise Elder. As more and more people shift their expectations and perceptions, becoming a healthy Wise Elder will be the goal of everyone.

15

TWENTY-ONE DAYS FROM ORDINARY TO REMARKABLE

LIFE'S JOB IS TO OFFER NEW CHALLENGES—TO ENCOURAGE OUR GROWTH AND CHANGE

According to psychologist Carl Jung, life offers new challenges in a seven-year cycle. A child begins school at seven years of age; experiences inner turmoil and hormonal changes at fourteen; faces career decisions as well as adult responsibilities at twenty-one; has a desire to settle down, have a family and "nest" at twenty-eight; begins to self-manage and transform uncomfortable, old, limiting habits at thirty-five; has a deep sense of unfulfillment or a sense of unrest and questions lifestyle and life direction at forty-two; and begins to make changes to lifestyle and emotional, physical and spiritual beliefs because of a mid-life self-management transformation at forty-nine.

By the age of fifty-six, spiritual matters, peace, love, calmness and wisdom begin to nurture the human spirit and become as important as physical wellness; at sixty-three, a late-life self-management transformation begins as retirement from full-time work is planned; at seventy and seventy-seven, challenges in education, career, marriage, having children, buying a home and saving financially are no longer preoccupations and the time has arrived for internal transformation to become a Wise Elder.

I also hold to this ratio of seven when I encourage a seven-day test-drive of my diet and a twenty-one-day potential transformation from ordinary to remarkable. Remember, it takes twenty-one days to downshift your taste buds back to their natural state of functioning.

YOUR EATING HABITS

The secret to feeling, thinking and living well is really no secret at all. By maintaining a vigorous energy system, detoxifying daily and staying emotionally balanced, you can function at optimum peak capacity all life long. With your new surplus of energy, revitalized cellular communication and motivation, you may even be able to repair other systems like your memory, hair, skin, vision, hearing or muscle tone, long thought to have deteriorated beyond repair.

Researchers and scientists have seen in their laboratories the amazing results I am talking about. It never ceases to amaze me when over and over again, on a daily basis, I see these remarkable transformations in so many people. I have seen people from twenty-four to eighty-four years of age regain their youthful vigor and well-being. They are rejuvenated! If you follow my simple recommendations, you will boost your body's ability to fight cancer, heart disease, Alzheimer's, depression and memory loss and keep yourself in a low-risk category for disease. You will never regret it, not even for a moment.

However, the changes in diet and lifestyle required to accomplish the transformation from ordinary to remarkable cannot be realistically achieved overnight; instead, they must be introduced slowly, one step at a time, over a twenty-one-day cycle. The good news is that it takes only minor adjustments in your current eating pattern and lifestyle to produce dramatic improvements in your energy, mood, enthusiasm, happiness and contentment. Even if your diet and lifestyle require a major overhaul, the process can be relatively painless and give you a "home-court advantage."

OUR CHILDREN'S EATING HABITS

I am especially concerned about the eating habits of our children, because these habits often persist throughout life. I am also aware that unless healthy food meets the new standards of taste and convenience, children may not eat it. Therefore, I encourage you to make healthy food fun for your children. Your children are in a state of perpetual motion. Their energy production mechanisms are in high gear, but the fact that they can seemingly run on empty is deceptive. It is easy to teach them to eat at regular times when they are hungry and not just because they are bored or upset. Keep healthy food in your house.

Think of healthy nutrition as the ultimate form of preventive medicine.

The *Journal of Pediatrics* in April of 2005 reported on a study of the daily sugar consumption of five thousand children aged two to five. The disconcerting results revealed that in two- to three-year-olds, average sugar consumption is 14 teaspoons a day and jumps to 17 teaspoons daily (mostly from pop) in four- to five-year-olds.

Help your children develop the lifetime habits that will prevent them from suffering a system-wide energy crisis, a life-threatening illness or an emotional meltdown in their adult lives. In the short run, it is all about them looking and feeling terrific—not just on good days, but every day. In the long run, it is about maintaining their bodies' master energy system on which their future bodies, emotions, motivation and brainpower depend.

Karen Corley, my dedicated research assistant, is the mother of four healthy, happy boys. Recently, she made this statement: "Remember that your children trust you and that includes the foods you give them. Know that your child's health is in your hands and that your biggest gift, next to love, is a lifelong habit of healthy eating." She continued on to say, "As a mother I have the responsibility of making healthy food choices for my family and presenting them in a way that appeals to everyone's personal needs. It has been a joy to see my children thrive and have natural, unprocessed foods and supplements be an everyday part of their lives."

The Best Time to Prevent Cancer and Heart Disease Is Fifty Years Before It Begins

Several human studies have found a link between fetal exposure to contaminants and toxins and illness in young adults. Several studies reviewed showed the correlation between secondhand cigarette smoke and childhood asthma, pneumonia and bronchitis; pesticides, paints, paint thinners, solvents and household cleaners and leukemia; and parents' occupational exposure to toxins and brain dysfunction leading to ADD (attention-deficit disorder) and ADHD (attention-deficit hyperactivity disorder) in children.

An embryo and fetus develop at a much faster rate than an adult. While this development occurs, cell division and growth is rapid. These rapid changes provide many opportunities for mistakes to occur. If a fetus is exposed to several toxic compounds, changes may occur that directly cause cancer or lengthen the period of sensitivity to carcinogens, therefore making the child more susceptible to cancer later in life. Feed both yourself and your baby cell-friendly foods and moods, so they will love you back for a healthy, energetic lifetime.

BETTER EATING BASICS

Eating right will produce better energy results and balanced moods quickly. Follow the guidelines listed for each week, and maintain the previous week's recommendations as you progress. In Week 3 you will still be doing what you learned in Weeks 1 and 2. By Week 3 you'll have developed an essential base of energy-eating and mood-balancing habits. Remember, there are only three essential food groups: protein, fat and carbohydrates.

Week 1: Get Energized

Do not skip breakfast. Make it a power protein shake and include berries. Follow one basic rule diligently: Never eat a meal without lean, high-quality protein and always eat your protein source first. Your protein source may be lean animal-based protein or lean plant-based protein. Drink two full glasses of water before breakfast, two more mid-morning, two more mid-afternoon and two more by 7:00 p.m. Eat all the salads and vegetables you want at lunch and supper and remember to include your protein. Eat two pieces of colorful fruit daily! Eat all your food sitting down, enjoy chewing, and savor your food.

EAT YOUR PROTEIN SOURCE FIRST AT EACH MEAL

"Protein" comes from the Greek root meaning "first." It may seem odd at first to eat your fish, tempeh or chicken before your salad, but doing so will ensure that you will avoid a glycemic reaction. Note that:

- It takes twenty minutes for your stomach to make the "I'm full" hormone cholecystokinin (CCK), the "stop eating" hormone GLP-1 and the "brain-energizing" hormone glucagon, so eat slowly.
- You can use a little fresh lemon juice, fresh lime juice, apple cider vinegar or fresh cinnamon sprinkled on any food, as this also helps you avoid a glycemic response and keeps insulin blood levels steady.
- Your appetite will be satisfied for four full hours.
- Every meal should have some healthy fat so the "I'm full" hormone leptin is elevated.
- "In many female patients I have seen long-term protein starvation lead to loss of face and body skin tone," writes Dr. Nicholas Perricone in *The Perricone Prescription.*

A Word About Eating Salmon

EAT WILD, NORTHERN B.C. AND ALASKAN SOCKEYE SALMON

Wild, British Columbian and Alaskan sockeye salmon are the most abundant and treasured of the wild Pacific salmon species. They have a deep red flesh and, of all wild salmon, have the highest concentration of omega-3 essential fatty acids and the biological antioxidant astaxanthin. Studies suggest that astaxanthin is ten times more effective as an antioxidant than other carotenoids, and one hundred times more powerful than Vitamin E. This natural pigment, which gives sockeye its rich color, comes from their diet of marine algae, zooplankton and krill. Because sockeye live only about four years and eat primarily a vegetarian diet, they are less prone to accumulate harmful contaminants than are other species. Studies have shown that wild, northern B.C. and Alaskan sockeye salmon are among the purest fish ever tested. Salmon is heart healthy.

British Columbian sockeye salmon is available canned and, increasingly, fresh and frozen as its unique characteristics have contributed to its growing popularity. When cooked or processed, the deep red flesh retains its color to a higher degree than that of other salmon. Sockeye is a rich source of the "brain smart" DHA and "mood smart" EPA fats, and has firm flesh as well as a full, delectable flavor. The B.C. sockeye's color, firmness, flavor and nutritional profile make it one of the most desirable of all wild salmon species and an energizing cell-friendly food. Salmon is a rare dietary source of dimenthylaminoethanol (DMAE.)

YOUR BEST PROTEIN SOURCES

Best Choice Proteins	Fair Choice Proteins	Poor Choice Proteins
Vegetarian		
hemp protein powder	roasted seeds	salted, roasted seeds
soy protein powder	roasted nuts	salted, roasted nuts
tofu, extra firm	plain almond butter	salted almond butter
tempeh, natto, miso	plain peanut butter	salted peanut butter
edamame		
soy beans		
legumes		
macadamia nuts		
raw, unsalted seeds		
raw, unsalted nuts		
Meat & Poultry		
(free range & grass fed)	beef, lean cuts	bacon
pork, lean cuts		hot dog
chicken breast, skinless		pepperoni
turkey breast, skinless		pork sausage
lamb		salami

Best Choice Proteins	Fair Choice Proteins	Poor Choice Proteins
Fish		
sardines calamari anchovies halibut salmon snapper mackerel	albacore tuna, canned in water shrimp scallops lobster clams	tuna, in oil
Eggs		
eggs from free-range, organic, vegetarian-fed chickens	eggs from vegetarian-fed chickens	eggs from animal-fed chickens
Protein-Rich Dairy		
whey isolate protein powder cheese, low-fat cottage cheese, low-fat yogurt, plain, low-fat organic milk, low-fat mozzarella, skim ricotta, skim	mozzarella ricotta hard cheeses milk, 2 percent	processed cheeses whole milk

A Note on Eggs: In 2001 the American Heart Association exonerated eggs—they are back to being a good food. Three poached eggs provide 840 mg of tyrosine and 24 g of protein.

Fresh salmon contains dimenthylaminoethanol (DMAE), which dramatically boosts brainpower. DMAE is also found in high levels in anchovies, sardines and mackerel and is naturally produced in the human brain. Europeans call sardines and anchovies brain food.

DMAE primarily boosts the production of acetylcholine, a crucial neurotransmitter responsible for carrying messages between brain cells, and from the brain to the muscles to control body movements. DMAE causes a noticeable boost in the ability to concentrate and focus, and significantly improves ADHD-related diagnosis.

Acetylcholine is also involved in higher brain functions like learning, recall, improved focus, mental clarity, brainpower, good moods and both memory ability and potency.

HOW MUCH CONCENTRATED PROTEIN IS ENOUGH AT ONE MEAL?

- 2 scoops of whey isolate protein powder or 4 scoops of hemp protein powder (24 grams of protein)
- 3 eggs (24 grams of protein) from free-range chickens fed flax seeds
- 1 cup of dry curd cottage cheese (20–30 grams of protein)
- 2 cups of beans or legumes, especially edamame (25 grams of protein)
- a 6 oz serving of pasture-fed meat, poultry or wild fish, approximately the size of the palm of your hand (20–30 grams); wild game is especially lean and rates high

Combining Protein with Carbohydrates for All-Day Energy

One important consideration is to always eat some protein at each of your three meals. Protein consumed with a carbohydrate food will lower the glycemic index of the carbohydrate and slow down its rate of digestion as the protein slows the breakdown of that food to glucose (blood sugar). This prevents a sharp rise in insulin levels and gives you robust, all-day energy. Whey isolate protein powder boosts glucagon-like peptide 2 (GLP-2) levels—a regulator of nutrient absorption that also maintains intestinal lining.

REMEMBER THIS IRREFUTABLE FACT

Your body cannot store protein. If you want high-quality, toned, supple skin, hair and muscles, you need to eat lean protein daily. You must have protein at each of your three meals every day for glowing skin, strong, lean muscle mass and stable insulin levels for constant abundant energy and superior good moods.

Week 2: Eat More Frequently

Eat three meals and two snacks and spread them throughout the day. Instead of breakfast, lunch and supper, eat:

breakfast	7:00 a.m.
mid-morning snack	10:00 a.m.
lunch	12:00 p.m.
mid-afternoon snack	3:00 p.m.
supper	6:00 p.m.

Do not eat after 8:00 p.m., except on special occasions. It takes one hour to begin to digest foods and for the next three hours, sugar (glucose) from digesting food enters your bloodstream and causes the sugar-storage hormone, insulin, to rise or spike. Insulin is a powerful brute of a hormone and when it rises, it reduces the levels of your sleep hormone, melatonin. Depressed melatonin levels mean you will not get a deep, regenerative sleep and will feel groggy in the morning.

BE PART OF THE SOLUTION

Every day, detoxify and cleanse endotoxin metabolic waste and exotoxin-intruding chemicals and pathogens from your body for good digestion and absorption, enhanced brainpower and more dynamic energy. Use a detox formula specifically designed to safely and deeply clean your liver, kidneys, blood and skin to eliminate exotoxins, called xenobiotics, like alcohol, pesticides, preservatives, insidious trans fats and chemical pollutants before they harm your faithful cells. *Xenos* is the Greek root for "foreigner"—xenobiotics are foreign, invading chemicals. A daily detox improves digestion and absorption of critical nutrients in your intestines and is a wonderful way to avoid unpleasant cleansing crisis reactions like headaches, nausea, rashes, pimples or diarrhea. A good detox formula will be strong enough to be effective, yet gentle enough to avoid a cleansing crisis. It will also improve your overall health and help you control your weight.

Week 3: Change Your Carbs to Natural

The easiest guideline that I can give you is to choose carbohydrates that are closest to their original form. You need lots of very low-density carbohydrates (vegetables, salads, berries) and a moderate amount of low-density carbohydrates (fruit). They are low on the glycemic index. Very low-density vegetables, salads and berries give off their energy source, glucose, very slowly as it untangles from the fibers. Low-density fruits do the same, and I recommend that you eat only four to six servings of colorful, fresh fruit or melons daily. A serving size is considered half a cup. Vegetables are about 30 percent fructose, fruits are about 70 percent fructose and grains and starches are 100 percent glucose.

CHANGE YOUR CARBS TO NATURAL

Original Source	Good Source	Poor Source	Processed
whole grains	whole grain bread, pita, pasta	white bread, pasta	cheese-flavored crackers canned pasta
potatoes	baked potatoes mashed potatoes with skins	French fries	potato chips instant mashed potatoes
rice	whole grain brown or red rice	white rice	puffed rice cereals
apples	apples, dried apples	refined, sweetened apple juice	apple strudel
oats	whole oat oatmeal	instant oatmeal	oatmeal cookie

YOUR BEST CARBOHYDRATE SOURCES

Best Choice	**Fair Choice**	**Poor Choice**
Very Low-Density Carb	***Low-Density Carbs***	***High-Density Carbs***
all berries	oranges	corn flakes
cherries	bananas	puffed wheat
plums	apricots	rice cakes
prunes	papaya	French bread
grapefruit	mango	instant rice
chestnuts	grapes	instant potatoes
yogurt, low-fat	whole-grain pasta	ice cream
peaches	multi-grain bread	pop
apples	lentils	white rice
pineapple	peas	corn chips
pears	pinto beans	bagels
all vegetables	navy beans	muffins
all salad greens and sprouts	chick-peas	bakery items
all herbs and spices	rye crisps	alcohol
		dried fruit

FRUITS AND THEIR SUGARS

Fresh Fruit to Eat	**Grams of Sugar per 100 Grams**
grapes	18.1
banana	15.6
mango	14.8
cherries, sweet	14.6
pineapple	11.9
apple	11.9
pear	10.5
blackberries, blueberries, raspberries	8.0
Dried Fruit in Moderation	
dates	64.2
figs	62.1
raisins	62.0
prunes	44.0
apricots	38.9

continued

Sugars in Moderation	Grams of Sugar per 100 Grams
sucrose (table sugar)	97.0
brown sugar	89.0
maple syrup	85.2
honey	81.9
molasses, blackstrap	60.0

RATE YOUR ENERGY AND HUNGER 3 HOURS AFTER YOU EAT

Is Your Protein-to-Carbohydrate Ratio Correct?

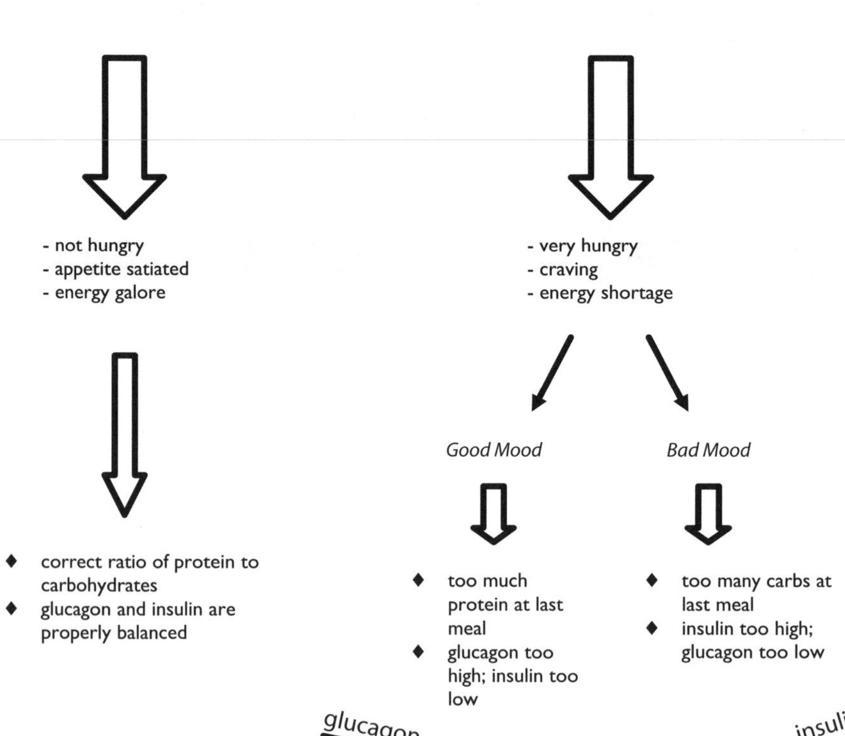

You absolutely need healthy fats every day. Your brain is 60 percent fat. Some dietary fats are more desirable than others. Marianne Leblanc, MD, recommends reducing saturated fat to no more than 3 percent of calories—no more than 6 grams on two thousand calories a day.

YOUR BEST FAT SOURCES

Good-for-You Fat Sources	Use Sparingly—If at All
wild triple fish oils for EPA and DHA	salted, colored butter
extra virgin olive oil	sour cream
high-lignan flax seeds, ground fresh	full-fat cheese
hemp, sesame, sunflower and pumpkin seeds	fried foods
borage, black currant or evening primrose oil	commercial baked goods
macadamia nuts	potato chips
unsalted raw nuts, e.g., walnuts and almonds	salted, roasted nuts
avocado	salted, roasted seeds
almond butter	sugary peanut butter
organic peanut butter (afloxin free)	partially hydrogenated oil
organic coconut oil as a butter	French fries
unsalted organic butter	sweetened yogurts
high-lignan flax oil in strict moderation	processed meat slices

Note: Omega-3, -6 and -9 fatty acids are already part of your health routine, but don't forget omega-7 fatty acids from eating just six to ten macadamia nuts a day or 1/8 tsp of sea buckthorn oil derived from the fruit and seeds. Omega-7 fats nourish delicate body tissues like the skin and the membranes that line the digestive and urogenital tracts.

WHERE TO FIND YOUR BEST FAT

For	Daily Source
lignans and short-chain omega-3 fats	2 tablespoons of both flax and sesame seeds ground in a coffee grinder and added to your breakfast protein shake
long-chain omega-3 fats	1 softgel of enteric-coated triple fish oils, high in "mood smart" EPA and "brain smart" DHA at breakfast, lunch and supper
biologically active preformed omega-6 fats, the precursors to gamma linolenic acid	1,200 mg of borage oil contained in three fish oil softgels *or* ½ teaspoon of borage oil *or* ¾ teaspoon of blackcurrant seed oil *or* 1,000 mg of evening primrose oil
omega-7 fats	6–10 macadamia nuts (or ⅛ tsp sea buckthorn oil)
omega-9 fats	2 tablespoons of organic extra virgin olive oil on your salads or vegetables

Sample Meals

Breakfast

Power protein shake:

- 8 oz of water or hemp, rice or fat-free milk
- 2 scoops high-alpha whey protein powder
- 3 huge tablespoons of unsweetened fat-free yogurt
- 2 tablespoons each of ground flax and sesame seeds
- 1 cup of fresh or frozen berries
- ½ teaspoon of borage oil

Note: Blend for only 10 seconds in blender.

Take 1 capsule of enteric-coated EPA and DHA wild, triple fish oils.

535 calories, 35 g protein, 60 g carbs, 12 g fat

MID-MORNING SNACK

1 piece or cup of fresh fruit like colorful berries, melon, black cherries, apple, pear or papaya

100 to 200 calories

Three Lunch or Dinner Suggestions

6 oz (raw weight) skinless chicken breast/grilled *or* 2 tempeh patties
1 medium baked yam topped with salsa
4 cups mesclun salad with olive oil dressing
2 cups of carrot, celery or red pepper sticks
1 cup radish, garlic, broccoli or sunflower sprouts
600 calories, 35 g protein, 85 g carbs, 15 g fat

* * *

½ cup old-fashioned oatmeal
½ cup fat-free milk or rice/soy/hemp milk
1 tablespoon hulled sunflower seeds
1 tablespoon each of raw almonds and walnuts
1 tablespoon each of hemp seeds and sesame seeds
6 macadamia nuts
½ cup of fresh or frozen berries

cinnamon to taste
(add nuts and seeds once oatmeal is cooked)
500 calories, 20 g protein, 60 g carbs, 20 g fat

* * *

6 oz fresh, wild salmon broiled *or* 2 cups boiled edamame legumes with lemon juice, dill and tarragon
2 cups steamed orange squash with saltless seasoning
2 cups raw grated carrots, beets and turnips
½ baked potato topped with salsa or 2 teaspoons butter
500 calories, 25 g protein, 70 g carbs, 22 g fat

MID-AFTERNOON SNACK
handful of unsalted, raw seeds or nuts
200 calories
or
2 hard-boiled eggs
100 calories

WHAT IS ON YOUR PLATE MAY HELP TO SAVE YOUR SIGHT

Please don't forget about your eyesight. According to the National Eye Institute, more than 45 million North Americans suffer from cataracts, Computer Vision Syndrome (CVS) and the irreversible effects of age-related macular degeneration (AMD), the leading cause of acquired blindness in North America. A study recently released by the University of California, San Diego Shiley Eye Center, and published in the Archives of Ophthalmology, supports the idea that macular degeneration, cataracts and CVS patients benefit from self-management training, with special emphasis on controlling their diet. Leading eye experts say that preserving your vision begins with what's on your plate.

1. Lutein and zeaxanthin are two of the seven hundred plant pigments called carotenoids that give plants their colors. Load up

on lutein- and zeaxanthin-rich foods, such as eggs, dark green leafy vegetables, and salads. This will significantly lower the risk of eye-related macular degeneration. Lutein in eggs is up to 300 percent more bioavailable than vegetable sources of lutein. Lutein and zeaxanthin provide the yellow pigment found in these foods and help protect against AMD by blocking harmful blue light from reaching and damaging the cells in the central retina of the eyes, causing blurred or fuzzy vision starting in our forties or fifties.

2. Take an antioxidant supplement. A National Eye Institute study found that those with AMD who took a daily antioxidant supplement containing a minimum of 160 mg of vitamin C, 30 IU of vitamin E, 3000 IU of beta carotene, 10 mg of co-enzyme Q10, 15 mcg of selenium and 15 mg of zinc reduced their risk of developing advanced AMD by 25 percent and the associated vision loss by 19 percent. Nerve cells must have selenium to produce glutathione, one of the eye's most important antioxidants.
3. Pack in the produce. Fruits and vegetables are filled with beneficial phytonutrients that help to prevent oxidation. They also help you achieve a healthy weight because they fill you up on fewer calories. The National Cancer Institute recommends that adults eat five to ten servings a day.
4. A compound called A2E builds up in the retina and ignites when light in the blue spectrum reaches it, causing severe free radical damage to the eye. In 2004, *Carcinogenesis Journal* discovered that a bilberry extract containing at least 10 mg of a polyphenol called delphinidin stops A2E oxidation and furthermore prevents formation of cancerous tumors by inhibiting activator-Protein-1, which is an enzyme that cancer cells use to proliferate.
5. Get moving. The National Eye Institute says that individuals with early signs of potential AMD, cataracts and CVS who exercised three times per week were 25 percent less likely to get AMD compared to non-exercisers.
6. The Age-Related Eye Disease Study of 4,513 participants reported that AMD was significantly decreased by 53 to 60 percent in those people who had the highest intake of the omega-3 fatty acids from fish oils, EPA and DHA. In particular, DHA is selectively absorbed and retained in the photoreceptors of the eye.

REJUVENATE YOUR BRAIN: EAT BERRIES DAILY

Can you repair and restore the brain's broken and dysfunctional circuits and cell signalling or communication pathways once some of its function has been lost? The answer is a resounding *yes*!

In 1999 and in a 2003 follow-up study, Dr. James A. Joseph and researchers from Tufts University found that age-related brain degeneration could be delayed in young animals if they were supplemented with extracts of spinach and strawberries. This was a complete surprise because only strong experimental drugs were thought to be able to treat brain damage.

Dr. Joseph next experimented with blackberries and blueberries. He chose rats—equivalent in age to seventy-year-old humans—with age-related brain deficits that had diminished memory, an impaired sense of balance and motor-control decline. For eight weeks he fed the rats a regular control diet containing 1 to 2 percent of calories from either extracts of fresh blueberries, strawberries or spinach mixed with their regular food.

The totally unthinkable happened. The rats that were fed the strawberries, spinach or blueberries dramatically reversed their mental deficits, such as stroke and Alzheimer's. Their brains were operating and functioning at much younger levels—back to forty years of age from seventy—in relation to humans! Dr. Joseph was amazed by the results. He had rejuvenated old brains—yes!—with half a cup of berries. This is highly significant. You can reverse the tell-tale signs of brain aging and the insensitivity of receptors in the brain cells, and restore eroded integrity of the brain's circuitry to reverse dementia, short-term memory loss, the early stages of Alzheimer's disease and the degenerative decline in brain function.

Dr. Agnes Rimando, PhD, of the USDA's Agriculture Research Service recently discovered that berries contain a phytonutrient compound called pterostilbene that reduces elevated cholesterol levels more effectively than ciprofibrate, an anticholesterol drug. Eat one cup daily of fresh or frozen berries in your breakfast protein power shake. If you include "mood smart" EPA and "brain smart" DHA rich fish oils, the beneficial results are even better!

HERBS AND SPICES— NEARLY FORGOTTEN POWERHOUSES

Are you going to Scarborough Fair?
Parsley, sage, rosemary and thyme…
Remember me to one who lived there.
For once she was a true love of mine.

Medieval English folk song

Culinary herbs and spices are powerful, cell-friendly foods. Interestingly, the most overlooked part of almost everyone's diet is herbs and spices. Familiar culinary herbs and exotic spices have unsurpassed biomedical properties to heal, are incredible powerhouses to enliven food's color and flavor, and have unmatched antioxidant, phytonutrient and anti-inflammatory capacities. Herbs and spices enhance insulin sensitivity while decreasing cortisol levels.

Herbs

In 2001, the U.S. Department of Agriculture, working with Tufts University Sackler School of Graduate Biomedical Science, developed the oxygen radical absorbance capacity (ORAC) scale to rate the ability of plant foods to neutralize the damaging effect of free radicals. Their research revealed that many common culinary herbs display more powerful free radical quenching or neutralizing capacities than blueberries. To learn more about herbs, I highly recommend Terry Willard, PhD's book *Encyclopedia of Herbs* and Dr. Hyla Cass's *User's Guide to Herbal Remedies*.

Herbs are fresh or dried fragrant plants used for medicinal purposes and to flavor foods. Spices are dried, aromatic plants used for medicinal purposes, to flavor foods and for food preservation. Rosemary is an excellent example of a spice. In Japan, researchers discovered that wild rosemary oil is four times as powerful as an antioxidant than BHT, the synthetic chemical commonly used to preserve food. Incredibly, garlic is rich in glutathione, allyl sulphides and other sulfur-containing compounds that strengthen the immune system and destroy cancer cells, microbes, fungi, yeast, and viruses. Oil of oregano is a super-tonic able to destroy fungi like *Candida albicans*, viruses like herpes, and waterborne parasites like giardia and cryptosporidium.

In Greek, oregano means "mountain joy," and oregano has the highest levels of the antioxidant polyphenols carvacrol, rosmarinic acid and thymol. To get the immense preventive, health power of oil of oregano and oil of rosemary, I encourage you to add them daily to your salad dressing.

THE ANTIOXIDANT CAPACITY OF FIFTEEN CULINARY HERBS OUT OF A RATING OF ONE HUNDRED	
1. Southwest oregano	92.18
2. Italian oregano	71.64
3. Greek oregano	64.71
4. Sweet bay leaf	31.70
5. Dill	29.12
6. Winter savory	26.34
7. Vietnamese coriander	22.90
8. Orange mint	19.80
9. Garden thyme	19.49
10. Ginkgo biloba	19.18
11. Rosemary	19.15
12. Lemon verbena	17.88
13. Sweet basil	14.27
14. Garden sage	12.28
15. Parsley	11.03

Use these culinary herbs liberally in your meal planning. Use fresh herbs, such as oregano, rosemary, dill, coriander, parsley, sweet basil, mint and thyme, in your salads. Use non-irradiated, organic dry herbs, such as oregano, dill, sage, mint, pineapple sage, chives, thyme and basil, on your vegetables. Add fresh herbs to all your cooked dishes to add unique flavors, medicinal healing and aroma and to aid digestion. Once hooked on indispensable herbs, you will want a backyard herbal garden, or a large pot or window-box garden of fresh herbs. I do all three… bon appétit!

Spices

Today, spices remain as important to daily well-being as they did to all the early explorers, navigators and trade merchants who plied the high seas in the wealthy trade of exotic culinary spices. Even Christopher Columbus searched for a source of highly treasured spices. Do you use spices? Perhaps you use them more than you know: garlic and black pepper are a standard in most ethnic cultures' fine foods; cardamom, cinnamon, cloves and black pepper flavor chai tea; ginger, nutmeg, cinnamon and cloves are ingredients in pumpkin pie; ginger is instrumental in gingerbread, ginger carrots and Thai cuisine; turmeric, cumin, cloves, cinnamon, fenugreek, garlic and chillies are used in curry; cardamom, allspice and cinnamon are elements in apple pie; cloves are used in deodorant; eggnog contains nutmeg; and black pepper, cumin, chillies and garlic are found in Mexican sauces.

Spices may be the most potent disease fighters available and can make your food choices delicious. Experiment with spices daily.

Spices to Use Daily

Black pepper stimulates hydrochloric acid secretion in the stomach to improve digestion and has potent antibacterial properties.

Cardamom is actually an aromatic herb that has antiviral, antibacterial, antifungal, anti-Candida capacities.

Cinnamon, especially Ceylon cinnamon, is a well-known medicinal spice. Cinnamon normalizes blood sugar levels—half a teaspoon a day reduces blood sugar levels in diabetics. Cinnamon can lower the glycemic load of any meal or breakfast protein drink.

Cumin contains anticancer, analgesic and anti-inflammatory properties. Cumin increases the liver's ability to support bifunctional Phase I and Phase II detoxification pathways.

Fenugreek seeds are used extensively in ayurvedic medicine to treat both diabetes and obesity. Fenugreek stabilizes high blood sugar levels and has antimicrobial and anticancer properties.

Ginger has amazingly effective anti-inflammatory capabilities. Ginger contains a polyphenol called zingibain that has almost 1,000 percent more protein-digesting power than papaya and is a common treatment for both rheumatoid arthritis and an upset stomach.

Turmeric is the famous, brilliant golden-yellow color in curry powder and the darling of medical researchers globally. Turmeric has been used for centuries in Chinese and ayurvedic medicine to treat gastrointestinal and inflammatory ailments. Turmeric and ginger work synergistically and are a much safer anti-inflammatory approach than aspirin and ibuprofen (standard nonsteroidal anti-inflammatory drugs, or NSAIDs). Turmeric, especially its curcumin polyphenol component, possesses unbelievable capabilities in the prevention and treatment of cancer as it arrests the growth of cancer cells at the G2 stage of their cell division. The journal *Prostate* (June 2001) cites research that curcumin inhibits proliferation and induces apoptosis (cancer cell death) in prostate cancer cells. The journal *Cancer* (September 2002) cites research that proves that curcumin inhibits pancreatic cancer tumor cell growth. Researchers at the University of California, San Diego state: "Curcumin should be considered as a safe, non-toxic and easy-to-use chemotherapeutic agent for colorectal cancers."

Curcumin lowers elevated homocysteine levels, a major risk factor for cardiovascular disease, and blocks estrogen-mimicking chemicals suspect in breast cancer. Curcumin shows dynamic promise to both treat and reverse the early stages of Alzheimer's disease. Curcumin stops progression of multiple sclerosis (MS) by reducing the production of the IL-2 protein, which destroys the myelin sheath that covers and protects most nerves like the covering of an electric cord. In MS the myelin sheath shreds or frays, exposing nerves and disrupting their cell-signalling effectiveness so messages are garbled and physical coordination declines.

Herbs and Spices That Do Better in Capsules

When you need a health boost, your herbs and spices have to be extra strong. In most cases, you just can't get a high enough dose from what's on your plate to give you the maximum health benefit.

1. **Garlic**: garlic, onions, leeks and shallots are members of the lily family that contain sulfur. Sulfur makes up 10 percent of the human body and is needed for clear skin and glossy hair and to build proteins. Allicin, a component of garlic, is an antiviral, antibacterial, antifungal agent, and it balances blood pressure. Use one capsule of aged garlic at each meal.
2. **Ginger**: for motion sickness, take 500 mg of the powdered extract 30 minutes before travelling, and then every 4 hours until the end of your trip.
3. **Oregano**: for cold sores, colds, the flu, parasites, or bacterial, viral or fungal infections, use oil of wild oregano rich in antifungal esters such as linalyl acetate and geranyl acetate. Use one to ten drops, four times a day, diluted in 2 ounces of water, or take capsules containing 450 mg of oregano three times a day.
4. **Peppermint**: a great stomach-calming herb or digestive aid. Peppermint oil, which comes in enteric-coated capsules, is one of the most effective treatments for irritable bowel syndrome (IBS). Three or four times a day, take one capsule containing 0.2 milliliters of peppermint oil with water before meals.
5. **Resveratrol**: a polyphenol found naturally in dry red wine. The Fred Hutchinson Cancer Research Center in Seattle discovered that red wine reduces prostate cancer risk by 50 percent in those who drank four to eight 4-ounce glasses per week. It also protects DNA from free-radical damage and protects cells from environmentally induced malignant transformation. Use 40 mg of resveratrol daily as a chemoprotective supplement.
6. **Turmeric**: Curcumin is the active ingredient in turmeric. It is used for powerful anti-inflammatory protection from the pain of osteoarthritis, rheumatoid arthritis and tendonitis and to protect both your heart and brain. As a blood-cleansing, anti-inflammatory, anticancer spice, use three 500 mg capsules, one at each meal, of turmeric.
7. **Capsaicin**: the active ingredient in red hot chillies, used successfully in painkilling creams and gels for muscle aches, arthritis and osteoarthritis. In May of 2005, an injectable liquid made of capsaicin became available. Initial test volunteers with severe osteoarthritis of the knee showed that five weeks after receiving a single injection, the patients were still pain free. This is a new alternative to injections of steroids.

Herbs and Spices Protect Against Cancer

Several commonly used culinary herbs and spices have been identified by the National Cancer Institute as possessing compounds that protect us against cancer. These powerful defensive herbs and spices include those belonging to the ginger, mint, garlic, parsley and turmeric families, as well as the potent flax seed we discussed in Chapter 7. They contain a diverse array of active phytonutrients (such as flavonoids, terpenoids, phthalides, and sulfur compounds) that can produce a serious defense against proliferating cancer cells.

Cilantro, Ginseng, Mint and Parsley

Cilantro, ginseng, mint and parsley are a good source of cancer-prevention phytonutrients. These herbs have beneficial substances that block metabolic pathways associated with the development of cancer, and help synthesize enzymes that metabolize and eliminate active carcinogens.

Terpenoids, the compounds responsible for the flavors of the mint family (basil, oregano, rosemary, sage, spearmint and thyme) suppress the growth of tumors. For example, rosemary and sage are abundant sources of ursolic acid, which inhibits cancer cell initiation and promotion.

In a large Korean study, those who had taken ginseng for one year had 36 percent less cancer that nonusers and those who used ginseng for five or more years had 69 percent less cancer. Ginseng extract was more effective than fresh sliced ginger or ginger tea in reducing the risk of cancer.

Garlic and Onions

In a large Chinese study, people with the highest intake of garlic, onions and leeks had a risk of stomach cancer that was 40 percent lower than those with the lowest intake. In an Iowa Woman's Health Study, consumption of garlic was associated with a 32 percent reduction in colon cancer. A Dutch study also revealed that stomach cancer occurrence in those consuming at least half an onion a day was about 50 percent lower that in those consuming no onions.

Ginger, Resveratrol and Turmeric

In 2003, researchers at the University of Texas MD Anderson Cancer Center in Houston revealed how various synthetic NSAIDs, such as aspirin and ibuprofen, as well as natural compounds, such as curcumin and resveratrol, inhibit tumor cell proliferation. Recently published in the cancer journal *Oncogene*, the study concluded that curcumin and resveratrol were among the most potent anti-inflammatory and anti-proliferative agents, while aspirin and ibuprofen were among the least potent. Scientists at Emory University in Atlanta, in 2005, showed that curcumin exhibited "a high degree of anti-cancer activity, preventing or interfering with angiogenesis," the process by which tumors supply themselves with nutrients that fuel their growth.

Clearly how we season our food affects our well-being. Salt, sugar and high-fat dressings may tickle taste buds, but they increase the risk of cardiovascular disease and cancer. Culinary herbs and spices give the very same satisfaction to food while providing a dynamic defensive measure of protection from cancer, a most dangerous foe.

Just five years ago, many researchers felt that herbs and spices belonged to the realm of folklore. Now, they are paying very close attention to the stunning and unprecedented discoveries of biomedical research findings that are registering a seismic scientific shock. Since the dawn of humankind, culinary and medicinal herbs and spices have been used for flavor, aroma, as food preservatives and for total life-supportive well-being. Their long-time use and medicinal application have proven not to be a myth, but a monumental truth.

16

IN PURSUIT OF HUMAN EXCELLENCE—MIGHTY BRAIN MESSENGERS

NUTRITIONAL NEUROSCIENCE

Nothing is more important to a successful and fulfilling life than an optimally functioning brain. Medical journals are full of news and discoveries of how to keep the brain at peak performance levels for a lifetime—from increasing the intelligence of fetal brains to preventing and reversing brain breakdown as we grow older. An article in *Psychology Today* in 2000 emphasizes that it is not idle speculation that we can prevent brain aging. The brain is even becoming the main focus of nutritional research worldwide. Nutritional neuroscience, as it is called, is barely in its infancy, yet every day it is producing some head-turning findings.

For the first time in our human history, science suggests that it is never too early or too late to increase brainpower, achieve and maintain a happy state of mind, and prevent or reverse brain deterioration like memory loss and the early stages of Alzheimer's and Parkinson's disease.

For years the brain has been the "forgotten organ," but ultra-fascinating nutritional neuroscience proves that the brain is always growing; it is an ever-changing complexity of cells, a miraculous organ malleable by internal and external influences. New technology allows neuroscientists to peer inside the brain as it is processing information, consolidating memory, learning, thinking and perceiving, and expressing depression, anger and even psychotic episodes.

NEUROTRANSMITTERS: MIGHTY MOOD ENGINE MESSENGERS

For the first time in human history, neuroscientists are understanding how profoundly you can influence the factors that control brain functioning through food, supplements, sleep, stress reduction, exercise and simple lifestyle changes.

It's almost mind-boggling to consider that brain chemicals, called neurotransmitters, zigzag and flash through brain neurons at speeds of up to 150 mph and lay down biochemical expressways, mapping routes that carry your every feeling and thought.

There have been over one hundred neurotransmitters identified, but most of them fall into four broad categories. The brain and body function optimally as a mind-body connection when the neurotransmitters are in balance or in sync. The four primary biochemical *mood engines* in our brain that actually define us as a particular personality are:

1. acetylcholine
2. dopamine
3. gamma aminobutyric acid (GABA)
4. serotonin

Each of us is a synergistic, biological entity composed of the interrelated systems of these four mighty neurotransmitters. This relationship between neurotransmitters; neuropeptides, their chemical messengers; and their neuronal cell receptors is responsible for human behavior (emotional moods, such as anger or pleasure); physical feelings (such as hunger or pain); movement (such as walking or running); involuntary processes (such as digestion and breathing); and cognitive abilities (such as intellectual understanding and memory).

Unless we intentionally increase our brain's neurotransmitters, we produce less each year after the age of thirty-four. Compounding the problem is the decline—both in number and sensitivity—of the billions of receptors that receive and transmit neurochemical messages.

All of us are dealt a genetic hand with certain physiological advantages and disadvantages. Our goal is to maintain our brain messenger advantages, while improving the brain messenger disadvantages—that is, maintaining a synergistic synchronicity, a mental, physical, emotional and spiritual balance. This is the formula for a happy, fulfilled, disease-free life as a Wise Elder.

Acetylcholine, the brain's memory architect, controls brain speed and ensures that both energy and information pass through each system easily. Acetylcholine controls creativity, self-esteem, insight, critical judgment, memory, language, spatial relationships, sensory impressions and interpretations, speech, reading and thought.

Stress and aging lead to a decline in the quantity of the enzyme choline acetyltransferase, which controls the biosynthesis of acetylcholine. Stress and poor diet cause an acetylcholine decline.

Full-blown depletion of acetylcholine results in Alzheimer's disease.

On April 7, 2003, the National Academy of Sciences established daily minimum requirements for choline, which is the building block for acetylcholine.

Adult men	550 mg
Adult women	425 mg
Pregnant women	450 mg
Lactating women	550 mg

Dopamine, the brain's energy revitalizer, controls energy release, energy consumption, drive and excitement about new ideas. Dopamine keeps us vigilant and alert, controlling the release of the red-alert hormones adrenaline and cortisol for the "fight or flight" response. It is also responsible for emotional drive and spontaneity.

Dopamine-producing cells are destroyed by environmental toxins, smoking or second-hand smoke, and poor lifestyle choices, such as alcohol and drug abuse or a junk food diet. Full-blown dopamine deficiency is known as Parkinson's disease.

GABA, the brain's calming mood regulator, is the brain's natural valium. It controls the brain's rhythm of thinking, talking and hearing, and provides genuine peace and calmness to your mind, body, emotions and spirit.

When GABA levels are low or out of balance, one experiences headaches, hypertension, anxiety, diminished libido and disorders of the heart.

GABA is involved in the production of the "feel good" neuropeptides, the beta-endorphins, which are produced after exercising or during times of deep prayer or meditation when you feel a quality of depth, blessedness, calmness and connectedness. GABA is a potent mood enhancer. In 2005, the journal *Audiology and Neurology* presented research that GABA allows nerve cells in the ear and brain to cross-talk more efficiently and improve hearing loss due to age-related hearing problems.

Serotonin, the brain's mood rejuvenator, influences appetite, cravings and obsessive behaviors. Low serotonin levels cause us to be impulsive, aggressive, anxious, restless and depressed and to exhibit compulsive habits including overeating and drug and alcohol abuse. Serotonin promotes equanimity, alert tranquility, confidence and a positive enthusiasm. Low serotonin levels create depression, which is often treated with the popular medications Prozac, Paxil, Zoloft and others known as Selective Serotonin Reuptake Inhibitors (SSRIs). These drugs inhibit the nerve cells from reabsorbing serotonin once it is released, thus prolonging the action of serotonin and giving short-term biochemical assistance. Low serotonin levels also cause PMS cravings and sleep disorders.

Pregnancy is an example of serotonin dominating other neurotransmitters. The "glow" that pregnant women have is largely due to increased levels of serotonin.

Melatonin, the hormone that puts you into deep sleep, is made from serotonin in a two-step process in the pineal gland in the brain. Serotonin is made in the brain during the day when you eat low-density, cell-friendly carbohydrates, and then gets rapidly converted to melatonin at sundown.

Unlike the other three major neurotransmitter groups, serotonin does not decline dramatically over time, although melatonin secretion declines sharply with age. But because the other neurotransmitters do decline after the age of forty-five, this creates an excessive dominance of serotonin over acetylcholine, dopamine and GABA. This dominance increases biological stress and cortisol levels, resulting in the blahs or "couch potato" syndrome, leading to anxiety, poor sleep, slower mental processing, impaired glucose metabolism and an energy decline, sexual dysfunction, poor balance and reduced impulse control.

THE 4 BRAIN LOBES AND THE DOMINANT NEUROTRANSMITTER

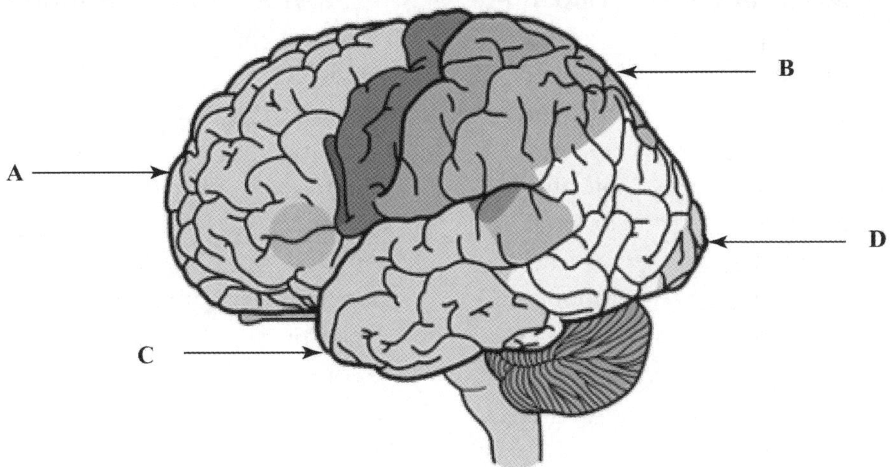

A) Frontal Lobe: Dopamine is the dominant neurotransmitter and controls the electrical circuitry of the brain for conceptualizing and long-term planning.

B) Parietal Lobe: Acetylcholine is the dominant neurotransmitter; is the thought, idea and intelligence center; and controls the signalling speed of brain transmissions.

C) Temporal Lobe: GABA is the dominant neurotransmitter and controls the brain's bioelectrical rhythm of sound processing, talking, thinking and acting.

D) Occipital Lobe: Serotonin is the dominant neurotransmitter and regulates visual processing, sleep and the brain's biochemical pace and mood.

RATE YOUR PERSONALITY DOMINANCE

Below are nine characteristics related to each dominant personality. Mark 5 beside those you feel are your dominant characteristics, 3 beside those you feel are moderate characteristics, and 1 beside those that are your weakest characteristics.

Acetylcholine		Dopamine		GABA		Serotonin	
caring	____	calm	____	loyal	____	able	____
creative	____	correct	____	dependable	____	adaptable	____
expressive	____	efficient	____	executive skills	____	calm in chaos	____
idealistic	____	goal oriented	____	hard working	____	curious	____
people person	____	objective	____	neat	____	decisive	____
romantic	____	original	____	practical	____	electric	____
spiritual	____	powerful	____	precise	____	flexible	____
trusted	____	rational	____	punctual	____	multitasker	____
unselfish	____	unique	____	realistic	____	welcoming	____
Total Score	____		____		____		____

Now you know your dominant character type and which neurotransmitter is dominant. The goal of the pursuit of human excellence is to merge and blend these personality characteristics at will, to grow and transform into a self-actualized human being, according to psychologist Abraham Maslow. A score of 140 or more indicates a self-actualized person.

NEUROPEPTIDES ARE "BIOLOGICAL CELL PHONES"

Your neurotransmitters, which contain the messages, use "biological cell phones" to send their intracellular communication over the microcircuitry of the brain's electrochemical web. Peptides and neuropeptides play an important role in mediating all messages over the electrochemical web, acting like a network of integrated high-speed computers.

Peptides are brain chemicals consisting of two or more amino acids held together by a peptide bond. Neuropeptides are peptides released by brain neurons as intracellular messengers in the vast, intricate and highly efficient communication network of our sophisticated brains. Scientific study of neuropeptides has only begun in the last ten years and neuroscientists are just beginning to unlock their secrets.

Neuropeptides are the biological cell phones that neurotransmitters and some hormones relay their messages with. There are no answering machines at neuron receptor sites receiving the messages, so neuropeptides have to be efficient because every biological cell phone call needs to be received and answered instantly.

All your fascinating neurotransmitter messages and genetic information are transmitted by neuropeptides. They decode, encrypt and transmit pain and forgetfulness, hunger and satiation, humor and cynicism, hope and hopelessness and energy and fatigue.

Neuropeptides can work for us or against us. For instance, you want to suppress the release of pro-inflammatory neuropeptides, the troublemakers, and enhance the production of anti-inflammatory neuropeptides, the super-helpers. Highly effective and multipurpose cell-friendly foods increase the production of good neuropeptides.

Neuroscientists are presently intrigued with and in awe of neuropeptides, which have remarkable potential for the brain and central nervous system, not just for transmitting emotions, sensations, intuitive thoughts, spontaneous insights and personality, but *consciousness itself*. A fight or flight response can be initiated in a matter of seconds, and its effects can dissolve in minutes. However, the true memory of that fear can last a lifetime. Decades later, you're still getting the same message. That is, the trauma of that fear will stay with you in your memory for years. Neuropeptides accurately decipher the coded message from the neurotransmitter, turn on the dedicated biological cell phone line and transmit it as a neurobiological sensation with the consistency of the most reliable computer.

Neuroscientists now track the hidden world of a whizzing neuropeptide as it moves at a millionth of a second, at lightning speed, at the mind's control. We don't need to listen as much for messages from outer space as much as we need to listen and respond to the bi-directional messages from inner space.

Consider sight. Close your eyes and recall a sight you once saw and really enjoyed. If you concentrate, you can envision that sight perfectly, flawlessly. The original sight was encoded on the neuropeptides in your brain, which carry and remember the conscious awareness of the moment and are able to recall it faithfully.

Neuropeptides convey the picture like a faithful camera, but, miraculously, they also encode the actual consciousness, feeling or emotion of the moment. What is joy? Neuropeptides celebrating because they have water, cell-friendly foods, and a lifestyle of deep sleep, laughter, exercise and enthusiasm. What is depression? Neuropeptides caught in deep sludge and uncollected trash, suffocating, being thrashed by free radicals, inflamed and exhausted with few available cellular receptors.

Every day, multiple neuropeptides are subjected to severe, damaging abuse from passing particles of chemical food colorings, sugar, trans fats, food preservatives, traffic fumes, second-hand smoke, stress, anxiety, guilt, regret, depressive moods, sleep deprivation, a lack of deep oxygenation and both exotoxins and endotoxins.

Exhausted neuropeptides give up easily, produce substandard performance, and decline in ability. If they are nourished, vitalized, cared for and appreciated, neuropeptides will flourish and convey emotions, feelings, information and intuitive thought effortlessly and faithfully. We need these neuropeptides so we can continue to learn, grow and transform.

If you want to function at peak performance, with synchronized, synergistic, balanced neurotransmitters and faithful neuropeptides that rejuvenate and revitalize with unprecedented success, you need to eat high-quality, natural food so you can enhance the natural, high-quality precision of your brain's electrochemical microcircuitry.

A LIFESTYLE TUNE-UP TO REPLENISH YOUR MOOD ENGINES

With no doubt, the most pervasive lifestyle issue today is acute stress. Fight it by replenishing your mood engines. Weight-bearing exercise boosts dopamine; swimming, biking, walking, running and aerobic exercises increase acetylcholine, GABA and serotonin; a nature walk enhances GABA; a game of chess or an interactive computer game replenishes dopamine; and writing a poem, letter or song restores acetylcholine. Foul language, loud, aggressive music and violent movies decrease production of acetylcholine, GABA and serotonin, but can overly raise dopamine levels so we seek more dangerous thrills. Electromagnetic currents from cell phones, old computers, televisions and microwaves may depress both neurotransmitter and neuropeptide efficiency and effectiveness. Radiation exposure from cell phones can be reduced to zero if you attach to your cell phone a ferrite bead; these magnetic beads are also used to stop data interference in computers.

Acetylcholine-Boosting Nutrients and Activities

To increase memory, focus, attention, learning and brainpower, you need:

- a phosphatide complex of 26 percent phosphatidylcholine, a direct bioavailable precursor to acetylcholine, which is found in cutting-edge "green drink" extra energy powders
- acetyl-L-Carnitine, which prolongs acetylcholine activity
- phosphatidylserine, which maintains neuronal membranes
- R(+)-lipoic acid, or R-dihydro-lipoic acid, which protect membranes from cortisol toxicity
- hyperzine-A, which prolongs acetylcholine efficiency
- alpha-glycerylphosphorylcholine, which helps boost acetylcholine

- acetylcholine-boosting foods: avocado, cucumber, lettuce, eggs, nuts, seeds, yogurt, organic dairy products, fish, fruits and vegetables
- acetylcholine-boosting activities: meditation, prayer, visual imagery, Tai Chi, Qigong, hatha yoga, rhythmic singing, rhythmic traditional dance and pleasing music

Dopamine-Boosting Nutrients and Activities

To increase your energy, enthusiasm, mood, creativity and motivation, you need:

- the amino acid tyrosine, which produces dopamine in conjunction with vitamin C, vitamin B6, taurine and glycine, combined with the herbs rhodiola rosea root extract, gotu kola and kola nut seed extract
- chromium, a trace mineral that augments dopamine
- dopamine-boosting foods that are rich in the amino acids phenylalanine and tyrosine: soybeans, edamame, walnuts, yogurt, wild game, rolled oats, wheat germ, seeds, eggs, cottage cheese, chicken and especially bioactive whey isolate protein powders
- dopamine-boosting activities: martial arts, tennis, swimming, walking, golfing, spinning, Pilates, aerobic exercises, weight-resistance training and mountain biking

GABA-Boosting Nutrients and Activities

To improve your calm, serene, alkaline and tranquil state of mind, you need:

- an alkalinizing, complete, cell-friendly, superabsorbable "green food" supplement
- inositol, a B vitamin that makes GABA
- the herbs turmeric, ginger and holy basil
- the amino acids taurine and glycine, which are GABA precursors
- N-acetyl-cysteine
- the family of B vitamins
- the amino acid L-theanine

- GABA-boosting foods: whole grains, legumes, vegetables, oranges, cantaloupe, nuts and mushrooms, especially oriental mushrooms like reishi and shitake
- GABA-boosting activities: reading, sitting in awe of nature, praying, meditation, deep breathing, meaningful pauses, hatha yoga and Tai Chi

Serotonin-Boosting Nutrients and Activities

To improve your good moods, joy, happiness, contentment and fulfillment, you need:

- high alpha whey protein powder
- St. John's wort herb, which boosts serotonin
- S-adenysol-L-methionine (SAMe), which acts in many people as a serotonin enhancer and natural antidepressant to enhance mood and alleviate melancholy
- folic acid, also referred to as folate or vitamin B9
- 5-HTP, which is an amino acid precursor to tryptophan, which in turn forms into N-acetylserotonin, then cascades into melatonin (for deep sleep) faster than the amino acid tryptophan itself
- serotonin-boosting foods that contain high amounts of the amino acid tryptophan: eggs, green vegetables, lean turkey, fish (like salmon), seeds, nuts and high alpha whey protein powder, hemp protein powder or soy protein powder
- serotonin-boosting activities: anything that resynchronizes the mind-body connection, such as aerobics to music, meditation, deep breathing, hiking, swimming, Tai Chi, Qigong, hatha yoga, tennis, volleyball, badminton, golfing, soccer and baseball

WHO ARE YOU?

Who are you? How does the world view you? Interestingly, the left hemisphere of the brain controls the movements on the right side of your body, and the right hemisphere controls the left side. Each person favors one side over the other, leading to predominant behavioral characteristics related to each side or hemisphere.

Dominant left-hemisphere individuals tend to focus on rational, systematic thinking, analysis, detail and accuracy. They rely on their practical skills to survive; they are ethical and prefer to be slightly introverted. Dominant left-hemisphere people tend to be very disciplined and well organized and are GABA dominant. GABA controls brain rhythm so these people have common sense, traditional values, integrity and thoroughness.

Dominant right-hemisphere people focus on intuition, feeling and aesthetics. They prefer to be outward. They are social, spontaneous, impulsive, creative, empathic and subjective. They have contagious enthusiasm and are sensitive to the feelings of others. Their predominant neurotransmitter is acetylcholine.

Today, you are the first generation ever to have the capacity to mix, merge and blend the best aspects of your left and right hemispheres—the right hemisphere's emotions and creativity with the left hemisphere's efficiency, memory and discipline. Unfortunately, wishing to do so is not enough, but eating three meals and two snacks a day of cell-friendly foods, practicing deep breathing to oxygenate brain tissues, taking therapeutic supplements and making lifestyle adjustments can do it quickly.

Neurophysician Eric R. Braverman refers to the personality and biological influences that each neurotransmitter has as a biotemperament, and states in his recent book *The Edge Effect* that "the problems and disturbances in our personality and emotional life are imbalances in neurotransmitters."

NEUROGENESIS AND CROSS-TRAINING FOR YOUR BRAIN

Mental aerobics can keep your brain cells healthy and help them to grow or regenerate. Dr. Elizabeth Gould of Princeton University has shown that laboratory animals continue to produce new brain cells in the hippocampus, the seahorse-shaped formation beneath the temples. Dr. Fred Gage and associates at the Salk Institute have shown that the brain can actually rewire itself and grow new cells for a lifetime, a process known as neurogenesis.

To grow your brain, like growing your muscles, requires cell-friendly foods, stress reduction and mental aerobics. Studies on mental aerobics have shown that the tasks must involve an element of effort.

You want to cross-train your brain so the left-hemisphere's logical analysis (reasoning, drawing conclusions), reading and writing, counting and math, and symbol recognition and information sequencing (organizing thoughts, making lists) will mix, balance and strengthen communication pathways with your right hemisphere, which likes to be involved in tasks such as emotional perception, a sense of humor, depth perception, dreaming, face recognition, artistic and musical activities, reading maps, finding ways out and staying oriented.

Your goal in mental gymnastics or aerobics is to build both sides of the brain, and alternate right-hemisphere exercises such as mazes and a sense of humor with left-hemisphere exercises such as logical and reading tasks. It takes seven to twenty-one days to noticeably improve or fine-tune overall memory fitness, creativity and learning capacity.

You need to create a mental cross-training routine to help build brain efficiency—to tone and strengthen your "brain muscles." No one form of exercise has been shown to be more effective than another, so use a wide variety of exercise choices to individualize your program. Work both sides of your brain and alternate your mental aerobic stimulation routine from right hemisphere to left hemisphere exercises.

Right- and Left-Side Balancing Exercises

Try using your non-dominant hand (i.e., your left hand if you are right-handed) in everyday tasks such as brushing your hair or teeth, or opening doors. Challenge your brain by reading a magazine, this book or a newspaper upside down. J. Robert Hather, PhD, in his book *The Brain Gate*, promotes his favorite memory strategy as look, snap and remember. Look at any object, take a mental picture, then close your eyes and think about all the details. Pay strict attention. Open your eyes and jot down some of those features. Improvement is remarkable in fourteen days. The accumulation of experimental evidence now proves that the left hemisphere is responsible for convergent thinking (the one unambiguous right answer) and the right hemisphere for divergent thinking (creative new possibilities).

Right-Hemisphere Aerobic Exercises

1. Mazes are great ways to train your visual-spatial skills.

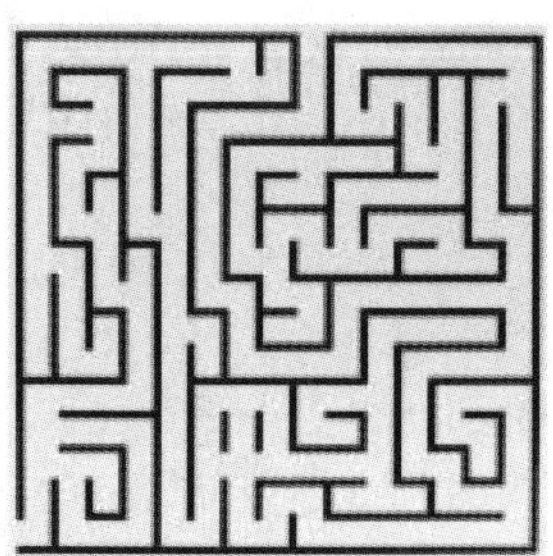

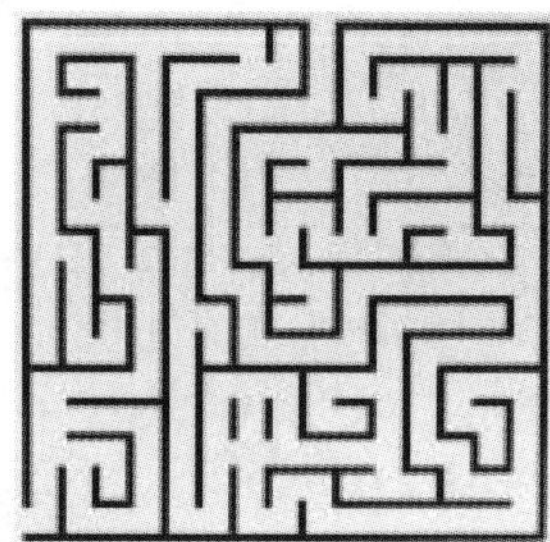

2. For each of the following, create a detailed, colorful vivid picture with great imagination and creativity: a dog, a car and a hat. Add interesting detail and specific designs, and think of various types of people and their personalities that may go with each one of these three words.

Left-Hemisphere Aerobic Exercises

1. Make a three-word sentence from the following jumbled letters: RYWOOAUEH?
2. Which is the odd one out? poodle, shepherd, black lab, Rhodesian Ridgeback.

ANSWERS: (1) HOW ARE YOU? or WHO ARE YOU? (2) shepherd is the answer since it can be something other than a dog.

Exercises to Enhance Overall Brain Function

- learn a new language
- do the crossword puzzle in the daily newspaper
- learn to paint, sculpt or do woodwork
- learn to play a musical instrument
- travel to foreign countries
- play card games, board games and some computer games
- take a computer class
- join an environmental group
- join a book club

- volunteer
- begin a daily exercise routine
- take dance lessons

Some occupations are primarily left hemisphere, such as accounting, law and mathematics. Other occupations are primarily right hemisphere, such as art, music and sports. The ultimate goal is to use both hemispheres to produce a superior type of learning referred to as whole-brain learning, strengthening the left and right hemispheres' wiring or neural mapping routes.

For additional cross-training exercises for both right and left hemispheres, refer to the recent book *The Memory Prescription* by Dr. Gary Small, Director of the UCLA Center on Aging, and his wife, Gigi Vorgan, available at www.drgarysmall.com. For a program to increase your memory, try Dr. Dharma Singh Khalsa, MD's Better Memory Kit. This kit is based on ten years of innovative, proven clinical methods to treat and reverse all types of memory loss, and is available at www.hayhouse.com. Abbie F. Salney, EdD, is the author and co-author of many challenging brain-building books, such as the *Mensa Think-Smart Book* and the *Mensa 365 Brain Puzzlers Page-A-Day Calendar* found at www.mensa.org.

THE POWER OF HUMAN RELATIONSHIPS AND THE STRENGTH OF SPIRIT

To ensure that our life has meaning, we need to put in place an overriding priority to pursue authentic meaning for ourselves. Our brain's neurotransmitters and neuropeptides function best when we attach great importance to human relationships, to tending and befriending others, and to other social and cultural concerns that give us genuine meaning and fulfillment. When you have meaning in your life, your body produces vast amounts of mood-modulating serotonin, which continues to filter out negative thoughts, feelings and impulses.

Furthermore, if we feel content that our life has meaning and fulfillment, once we go to sleep at each day's end our biochemistry will lengthen the duration of the important slow-wave or delta stage, the deepest most revitalizing phase of sleep. We influence our sleep patterns daily through our mind-body interactions, especially if we tend and befriend ourselves and others. This is why deep prayer, quiet reflection or meditation before we go to sleep is so immensely beneficial.

Shelly Taylor, a psychology professor at UCLA's Westwood campus, wrote a book called *The Tending Instinct*. She reasons that there are two options to handle stress: (**1**) you go to combat with it—fight or flight, or (**2**) you reach out to your support group and tend and befriend. Ninety percent of men fight or flee (the hormones cortisol and adrenaline dominate), and 90 percent of women tend and befriend (the hormone oxytocin dominates), since female responses have to incorporate the protection of offspring. The hormone oxytocin may need to be boosted if we are to become "survival of the wisest." Childbirth, breast-feeding, love, parent-child bonding, relationship bonding and the vivid memories of joy or loving times may well be the imprint of oxytocin combined with beta-endorphins. How do we raise oxytocin levels? We do so when we attach great importance to social and human relationships that enrich both ours and others' lives.

The next challenge is global wellness. These are worthwhile and achievable goals for everyone. There is really no other effective alternative.

17

IN PURSUIT OF HUMAN EXCELLENCE— THE MIND-BODY CONNECTION

We are like flowers: we are seeded, we grow, we blossom and give off our radiance, we start to dwindle and then we fade away. You have the potential to bloom and be radiant for much, much longer throughout your lifetime than you ever thought possible.

Dr. Hans Berger discovered that the human brain generates several distinct wave states, each associated with a certain state of consciousness. By changing the amplitude of each wave's threshold, you can change your internal mind-body communication frequency or state. This is the basis to biofeedback.

When the brain's low voltage energy communication patterns are recorded on an electroencephalogram (EEG), the brain waves resonate between 3.5 and 90 cycles per second. One cycle per second is called a hertz (Hz). All living organisms on earth have adapted to the underlying 8 cycles per second (8 Hz).

Back in Chapter 13, I told you that in the beta state, when your brain has a frequency of 13 to 39 Hz, you are fully alert and able to multi-task and produce at optimum, peak performance. In the alpha state, from 8 to 14 Hz, during normal waking hours, you are peaceful, assured, revitalized, focused and in a relaxed, calm, serene state of mind. In the theta state, brain waves are in the 4 to 7 Hz range and you are either in a state of creativity or deeply absorbed in prayer or meditation, and not aware of yourself, time or place. When reaching a meditative state, you gently slip from an alpha state directly into a theta state. In the slowest wave, the delta state, your brain has a frequency of 3.5 Hz and you are in deep, rejuvenating sleep.

> "I don't want to achieve immortality through my work...I want to achieve it through not dying."
>
> Woody Allen

Therefore, to keep your brain revitalized you need to meditate daily and sleep soundly—both good lifestyle choices for a biological cycle that allows you relief from the beta state or "acceleration syndrome," which makes you competitive and a successful multi-tasker. Staying in this acceleration syndrome, or the beta state of 13 to 39 Hz, for too long exhausts your mood-balancing serotonin levels and energizing dopamine levels, leaving your nerves frazzled and exhausted and prompting you to find a quick-fix stimulant such as caffeine, alcohol, "benzos," recreational drugs or prescription lifestyle drugs.

Modafinil, sold as Provigil (an abbreviation for "promotes vigilance"), is a lifestyle drug aimed at people who don't suffer from any diagnosable disorder. It sold US$200 million worth in the United States alone in 2004.

The cost of multi-tasking can be much less amusing when, for instance, you see someone efficiently chatting on a cell phone while driving, failing to notice the tractor-trailer turning and ending the conversation in a fatal accident. We must accept that the brain does have certain limits. Courses teach us to multi-task, but overall performance in each of the tasks is less efficient than if we performed each of them one at a time.

Recent research at the University of Wisconsin shows that more intense gamma waves (30 to 60 or even 90 Hz) mark complex operations such as critical memory storage and exceptionally deep concentration. Staying in this state, called gamma synchrony, helps to bind the brain's sensory and cognitive operations into the

1. Beta state: you are in the intense, multi-tasking 13–39 Hz frequency

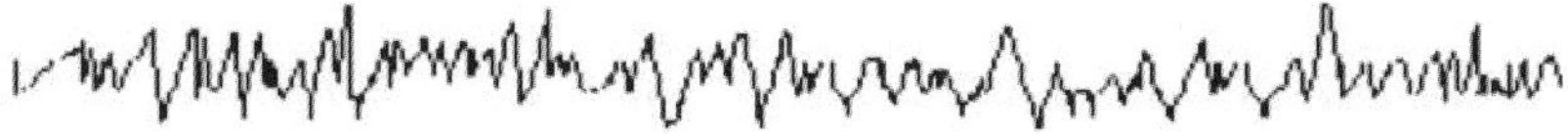

2. Alpha state: you are in the alert, restful 8–14 Hz frequency

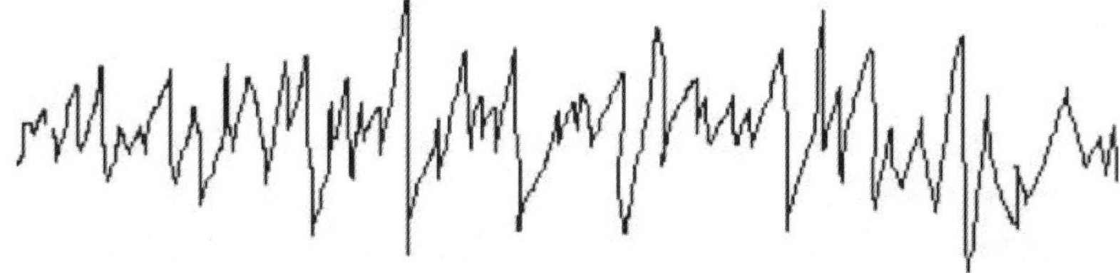

3. Theta state: you are in the serene, reflective and creative 4–7 Hz frequency

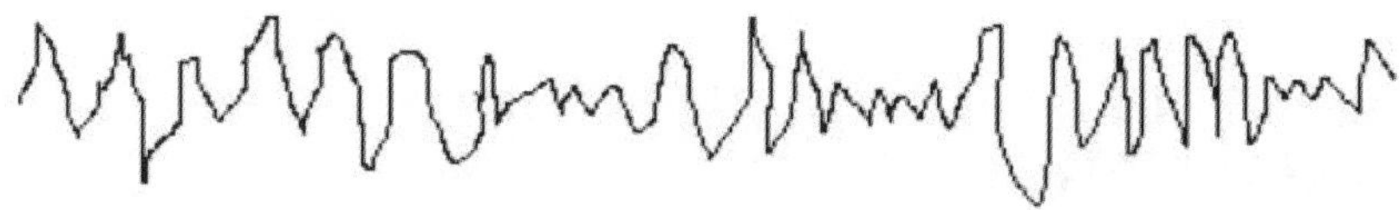

4. Delta state: you are in the deep, rejuvenating sleep 3–4 Hz frequency

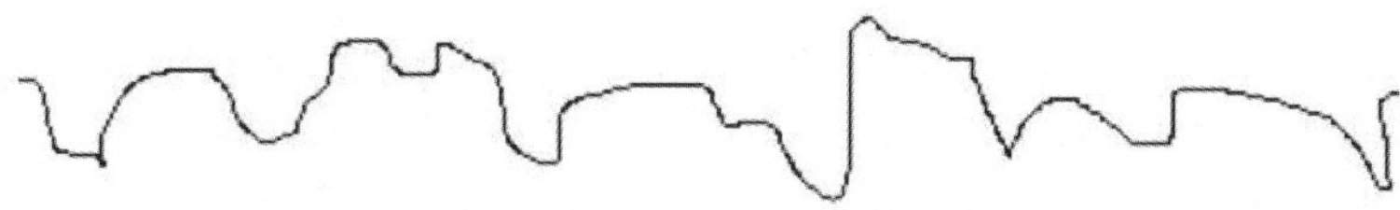

miracle of consciousness. Deep meditation or prayer, as well as listening to deeply calming music, can enhance gamma synchrony. A lack of gamma synchrony indicates discordant mental activity such as acute depression or schizophrenia.

Today you are bombarded with a wide array of human-made forms of electromagnetic (EM) radiation from cell phones, hair dryers, electric blankets and computer monitors. Your environment is also bombarded with radiation exposure from television and radio signals, satellite transmissions, radar signals and cell phone towers.

Although still very controversial, there is mounting evidence that continued exposure to such sources as 900 MHz (900 megahertz) cell phone frequencies can alter proteins in your cells and damage your DNA. Limit cell phone use or use a hands-free connection to limit radiation to your brain. In your car use an external antenna. It is the wire on your cell phone that acts as an antenna and concentrates the dose of radiation. As mentioned in an earlier chapter, you can clip on an inexpensive magnetic ferrite bead or choke to your cell phone line (antenna) to virtually eliminate radiation.

SYSTEM INTEGRATION—BI-DIRECTIONAL COMMUNICATION

The pineal gland in your brain, just behind the bridge of your nose, between your eyebrows, receives environmental stimuli of light and dark, and converts them into stimuli that communicate with your brain. Using light-dark sensory information in circadian rhythm, the pineal gland makes the hormone melatonin, which: (1) puts you into a deep, restful sleep, and (2) stimulates immune-boosting activity, as well as (3) being an antidote for stress by reducing elevated adrenaline and cortisol levels. This bi-directional communication is mind-body integration. Neuropeptides carry these messages between the environment and the brain and vice versa, often interchanging functional roles. An example is the neuropathway between the eyes and the pineal gland. Darkness prompts the neuropeptide called hypocretin (also called orexin) to convert light information to electromagnetic signals and turn on the pineal gland to produce melatonin, and daylight prompts the pineal gland to turn off melatonin production by using the bi-directional neuropeptide hypocretin.

HOW DARKNESS AND DAYLIGHT AFFECT PRODUCTION OF MELATONIN

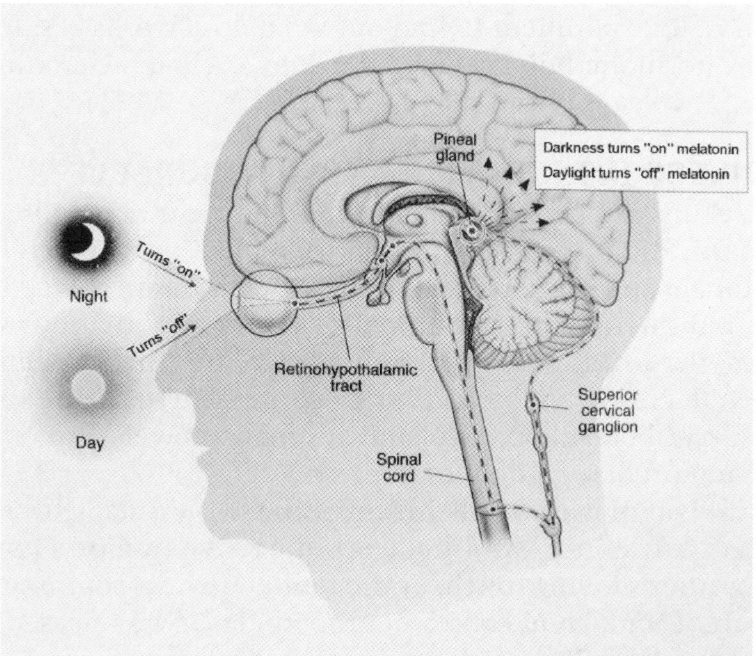

(Adapted from *The Scientific Basis of Integrative Medicine,* by Leonard A. Wisneski, MD and Lucy Anderson, MSW, CRC Press, 2005)

Melatonin

Because so many people use melatonin, I want to make a few notes on its use. Sleep is essential to good health, but 50 percent of North Americans over the age of forty have some form of sleep disturbance. Melatonin is a light-sensitive hormone secreted rhythmically as our biological clock—which is turned off by daylight and on by darkness—allows us to go into a deep sleep. From age forty on, melatonin production in the pineal gland becomes erratic; and by age fifty you produce only 50 percent of what you did at age thirty. Melatonin is inexpensive and widely available without a prescription. Your physician can test your saliva or blood to determine exactly how much melatonin you should take, if you need it. The rule of thumb with hormone replacement is to use the lowest dose that works. Start with 0.5–1.5 milligrams of pharmaceutical-grade melatonin taken sublingually because it is absorbed quickly. If you wake up frequently during the night, try time-released melatonin. You have to experiment to find out what dose works best for you. Take a "hormone holiday" each week by cycling melatonin—five days on, two days off.

SEAMLESS INTEGRATION—TRY IT YOURSELF

Touch your skin. Try it. Your brain and skin are using bi-directional communication. That is, your brain can tell if the touch is loving, affectionate and supportive, or if the touch is harmful, hurtful and painful. If the touch is affectionate, your central nervous system relaxes; the levels of cortisol and adrenaline (the red-alert hormones) decrease and you relax in contentment. If the touch is meant to inflict pain, cortisol and adrenaline levels soar, and you recoil and prepare to fight or flee.

"Survival of the wisest" means using this principle to full advantage. A friendly handshake, a supportive hug or a massage, your partner's loving touch, or the tender, loving, soothing caress of a parent for a child causes neuropeptides to be released in the brain, ignited by skin touch receptors that release other neuropeptides like beta-endorphins. These beta-endorphin neuropeptides send a healing, reinvigorating and positive message to the immune system, heart and brain.

> "It is confidence in our bodies, minds and spirits that allows us to keep looking for new adventures, new directions to grow in, and new lessons to learn—which is what life is all about."
>
> Oprah Winfrey

Studies in children's hospital wards and orphanages repeatedly demonstrate that babies and children deprived of human touch become ill, lose their appetite, lose weight and can cry more and suffer lifelong emotional damage. Babies and children who are held more, cradled and rocked will cry less and laugh more, and their immune systems flourish, their good moods get a boost and their health and well-being are enhanced for a lifetime. Just 15 minutes of daily massage help premature babies leave the hospital seven days sooner than babies who are not touched.

THE TALE OF TWO BRAINS

Yes, women and men's brains are different, but recent research uproots the old myths about which gender is good at exactly what. What is the latest science on the difference between women and men's aptitudes? There are several differences, many of which seem to change our behavior. Others don't. In the 1990s, neuroscientist Sandra Witelson of McMaster University's Michael G. DeGroote School of Medicine, in Hamilton, Ontario, became internationally known for her study of Albert Einstein's brain. She says, "the brain is a sex organ"; there is a variation between male and female brains.

In both women and men, daily brain patterns fluctuate and change within the same person. In fact, depending on your age, the time of day and your present circumstance, the changes within the brain vary greatly. The changes that occur in the brain when you are preparing for a final exam are vastly different than those that occur when you are lying comfortably in a hammock. From the time of conception your biology is constantly interacting with the environment—cross-talking—which makes life and the intricacy of human behavior very interesting.

Since the dawn of brain research, researchers have been intrigued by gender differences in the brain.

- In the late 1880s scientists said men were more intelligent because the corpus callosum, the bundle of nerve fibers that connect the two hemispheres of the brain, which was then considered key to intellectual capacity, had a greater surface area in men.
- In the late 1980s researchers said oops!—it is larger in women—and explained why the analytical left side of a woman's brain is more in touch with her emotional right side. In the late 1990s this theory was discredited.

- Most studies agree that men's brains are 10 percent larger than women's overall, even when the comparison is adjusted for men being 8 percent taller. But size of the brain does not predict intellectual performance. Amazingly so, most researchers cannot tell male and female brains apart just by looking at them.
- Women and men perform similarly on IQ tests.
- New brain-imaging technologies allow neuroscientists to map the living brain as it functions and grows with a great degree of accuracy and to move away from obsession over the size of the brain.
- Richard Haier, PhD, a psychology professor at the University of California at Irvine who studies intelligence, says that men and women have different brain architectures, and "we don't know what that means." In 2004, Haier and his associates administered IQ tests to a group of university students and, by analyzing scans of their brain patterns, discovered that parts of the brain that are related to intelligence are different between women and men. This was a major observation because for centuries, psychologists have assumed that all brains pretty well work the same.

Recent Observations

Women's brains are more interconnected, have more connections between the two brain hemispheres, and areas more densely packed with neurons than men's brains, and are perhaps better suited for higher diplomacy and social sensitivity. As women age, they keep more brain tissue than aging men in the front lobes of the brain, which are concerned with self-control, consequences and self-image. A female does her thinking, problem solving, and feeling in more parts of her brain than a male. Interestingly, women have fuller recoveries after a stroke than men and it is theorized that non-affected parts of women's brains compensate for injured neurons.

Men's brains are more compartmentalized, so men are more likely to say things without realizing how their actions will affect others in general and may not be as sensitive to high diplomacy. As most men age, they lose brain tissue in the front lobes of the brain that affect self-control, consequences and self-image. A male does his thinking, problem solving, and feeling in more focused, compartmental parts of the brain, so a stroke may incapacitate that particular compartment.

Women and men appear to handle emotions differently. The human brain processes emotions in a location deep within the organ called the amygdala. Women appear to have stronger connections between the brain's amygdala region and regions that handle higher-level functioning and language. This may explain why women are more likely to talk about their emotions and men tend to rationalize their emotions and carry on.

Since 1992, psychiatrist Jay Giedd, of the U.S. National Institutes of Health near Washington, has been using the MRI procedure to scan the brains of children. His research shows that most parts of the brain mature faster in girls, whose brain sizes peak around age fourteen to fifteen. Other researchers have shown that the areas involved in mechanical reasoning, visual depth perception and spatial comprehension appears to mature four years earlier in boys. Verbal language skills, handwriting, reading and recognition of familiar faces matured four years earlier in girls.

What Do the Gender Differences Mean?

So it really comes down to one question. How do we explain these gender differences? That is, how do we explain why most girls and women have better social sensitivities and verbal skills while most boys and men have better motor skills and mechanical abilities? Dr. Leonard Sax, a physician and psychologist, in his book *Why Gender Matters*, emphasizes that females can see patterns, texture and colors that men cannot see. They also hear and smell things better than men. Male and females who look at the same detailed landscape picture and report what they see report totally different things. He explains that in rats, for example, the male retina has more cells designed to detect motion. In females the retina has more cells built to gather information on colors and texture. Dr.

Sax suspects the same is true in humans, which explains why boys prefer to play with moving toys like cars, trucks and boats, while girls like to play with dolls clothed with colorful textures and draw with a wider range of colors.

Sandra Witelson, PhD, explains that some studies with baby girls show that they tend to give up and cry relatively quickly when faced with failure, while baby boys get angry and persist. She says, "What we don't know is whether that pattern continues into adulthood." Therefore, one easy solution for both males and females to overcome any biological weakness is the will, determination and motivation to repeatedly try a task until they master it.

A study in the journal *Behavioral Neuroscience* demonstrates that young, male rhesus monkeys proved better at finding food after they saw where it had been hidden, suggesting better depth and spatial memory. But, by maturity, male and female monkeys performed equally well, so aptitudes may not be the actual difference between males and females. Female monkeys dramatically improved their performance by practice and eliminated the early gender differences.

When I worked with teens at high risk, if they tried something not developmentally appropriate for them, such as mixing and socializing with high-achieving teens, they would, first, fail, and second, develop an aversion to that task or group of people. I noted that females were not achieving in the 1970s in engineering and computer sciences, not because they couldn't do it, but because they weren't motivated or taught properly. What does all this mean? What you believe yourself to be, you are—and will become. For instance, girls who are encouraged and motivated to achieve in math and sciences do just as well as boys. Today, 50 percent of all chemistry and biology bachelor of science degrees go to females, whose professors from an earlier generation are 60 percent male. Women have outnumbered men in college for more than a decade and more women than men graduate from most universities.

Researchers in Jokkmokk, an isolated town in the Swedish Lapland, have noted that girls consistently outperform boys in math and physics in Sweden. The difference is greatest in remote areas of northern Sweden. From a young age, boys focus on fishing, hunting, forestry and logging. Girls, meanwhile, want to move to the big cities in the south where they will need to compete for jobs in a high-tech society, so they focus on academics, stylish clothes, computer studies, social sensitivities and sciences. Leonard Sax, MD, is convinced that girls and boys have innately different learning styles and that in education we must change the environment so differences don't become limitations. Nora Newcombe, PhD, a Temple University psychologist who specializes in spatial reasoning, had males and females spend a couple of hours a week for ten weeks playing Tetris. Both males and females improved. She feels this means that if the males didn't train, the training females would outperform them.

Motivation

If we consider the rhesus monkey experiments led by Agnès Lacreuse, PhD, at the Yerkes National Primate Research Center, we can conclude that certain aptitudes may not be different between female and males. It may depend more at what stage in their life you test them. In elementary school, boys do not generally see, hear or listen as well as the girls. Therefore, they are more prone to become distracted, inattentive and bored. Perhaps boys need to sit at the front of all classes.

Many neuroscientists believe that the true gender gap is not about talent, but motivation.

Shirley Ann Jackson is the head of Rensselaer Polytechnic Institute. She feels that both genders need to see a career trajectory of someone of the same sex as them, which will demonstrate that with a dream, adequate skills, a commitment to success and relentless motivation, any job or career may be possible for either gender.

WHAT CONVERSATIONS ARE GOING ON INSIDE YOUR CELLS? MESSAGES FROM INNER SPACE

Organs, like our eyes, skin, heart and brain, are paragraphs that tell a story of their experiences to date. Tissues are sub-paragraphs that tell a more recent story about our life experiences. Cells are like sentences that tell us what is happening now! We cannot experience, or read, or alter these sentences as long as we are neurochemically imbalanced. This model of brain chemistry takes us above the discussion of "good people" or "bad people." We are physiologically and biologically all the same, though to different degrees we are consciously changing words and punctuation and adjusting the sentences in each cell with a greater sense of balance, especially neurochemical balance. The balance can be achieved only by using many of the progressive tools this book encourages you to keep in your genetic toolbox.

If the sentences in your cells are saying *we're tired; no way I'm exercising; I'll eat whatever I want; I feel lethargic; I really don't have the capability of destroying that cancer cell; I'll settle for mediocrity*; or *I'm stressed, anxious, or fearful of not succeeding*, they lose their lofty status and accelerate cellular communication breakdown known as mental or physical illness.

If the sentences in your cells are saying *today is a new day; I am full of potential for growth and transformation; I am equipped to deal with all the toxins that come my way; I feel radiant and energized; I feel great*; or *I feel compassion for myself and others*, they raise their lofty life-supporting values and accelerate communication fidelity known as mental and physical peak performance.

What conversations are going on in your 100 trillion cells? If you are caught in a biological cycle in which life-destructive habits give rise to destructive neurochemical events, you will continually reinforce those habits in self-perpetuating cycles by highlighting this mapping route. As an example, our brains have 100 billion neurons and a dense forest of communication pathways that send messages to receptor sites on cells. If we do the same action, eat the same food, crave the same sweet or stay in the same poor mood, then neuropeptides lay down familiar mapping routes or biochemical expressways in the brain.

We then are caught in our own repetitive negative behaviors that end up making us miserable, unbalanced and devoid of energy and that will eventually kill us. Stay depressed, lethargic, angry, anxious, craving, self-pitying, restless and shallow and you reinforce the neurobiological expressway that links up all the destructive connections and neurochemicals to keep you predictably locked in your increasingly addictive thoughts, feelings and experiences. Rationalizing merely keeps us from addressing the problem head-on. We then live lives of mediocrity. Eventually we pass on, having deprived ourselves of a life of fulfillment.

Amputees often experience sensations of phantom limbs moving, waving goodbye or shaking a hand. The brain is still following familiar mapping routes, communication expressways laid down in the brain over years of repetitive use before the loss of the limb.

CHANGE OR REARRANGE YOUR CELLULAR SENTENCES

Clinical studies and human experience suggest that neurochemical conditions can be changed or balanced, causing feelings, emotions and behaviors to change. Conversely, if you change a behavior, emotions and neurochemicals will change. This is the basis of the mind-body infinity loop. "Survival of the wisest" means using this bi-directional communication to become consciously aware, happy, alive, alert, loving and compassionate and co-creating our lives not just daily but from moment to moment. The wisest are rewiring and fine-tuning all their neurochemical expressways to maximize their happiness, health, emotional balance and spiritual maturity.

Scientists at UCLA discovered that when one of the lower-ranking monkeys begins to move up in the social hierarchy, their serotonin levels increase and they have better self-esteem and are more loving. Serotonin filters out negative feelings, thoughts and impulses. You can wisely raise serotonin levels while balancing dopamine and GABA levels. North Americans are running low on serotonin. Low serotonin levels cause dysfunctional regulation of the brain's centers of satisfaction and pleasure, which lead to cravings and addictive behavior to food, work, alcohol, drugs, gambling, abuse and aggression. We depend more now on anti-depressive medications, alcohol, drugs, caffeine, sweet treats and stimulants to temporarily raise serotonin levels so we can feel good about ourselves. All unnatural, addicting habits are becoming more and more socially acceptable.

Instead of patiently counselling many people who feel depressed or encouraging them to use diet and lifestyle techniques, doctors prescribe antidepressants, which are brain-altering medications designed to eliminate what might be uncomfortable but are a perfectly normal emotional response to life's challenges. If we experience low self-esteem or uncomfortable emotions and our serotonin levels or receptors decline, we can enhance their rate of recovery naturally.

If we medicate challenging neurochemistry, we may never have the capacity or opportunity to grow in love, compassion, acceptance and wisdom of the ages.

Our brains are like fingerprints; each of us possesses a unique neurochemical profile. We now have the technology in fMRI (functional magnetic resonance imaging) machines to map in 3D and interpret the overall pattern of brain activity. We can picture the topography—the inner landscape—of the brain actually thinking. Scientists have determined that you can use your own emotional genetic toolbox to intentionally generate different patterns of electrical and chemical activity—yes—to create better ones! The brain's neurochemical messengers have always played a silent but critical role in unfolding human history. Now you can actually enhance and boost their effectiveness in seconds—and the effects will last for decades.

We all know of many people who have made radical changes in their beliefs, outlook, diet, lifestyle and behavior naturally. Their serotonin levels rise, as do their self-esteem, social-esteem and love for themselves and others. Alcoholics, drug addicts and compulsive gamblers overcome addictions. They stop emotions and behaviors that are hurting them and others; many of these people begin whole new lives that are happy, fulfilled and life-supportive. People make dramatic changes in their perception of reality when they discover that their own underlying wisdom is fully capable and sufficient to support and nurture their human growth and happiness.

Your Neurochemical Profile

When we feel crummy, the hormone oxytocin floods our system like a wakeup call, trying to lead us to behaviors and emotions that will make us feel better. If we do not heed these signals, we can fall into depression, despair, hopelessness, anxiety and addictive behavior. People with good human relationships have higher oxytocin levels and do not stress out so quickly because they can recover quickly from disappointment or bad news. They have rewired their brains' neuromaps, and created new neurochemistry, new neurological topographies and new communication expressways that are no longer self-destructive but now are life-supportive.

These self-perpetuating cycles explain why being happy is really so much fun, and why depression can be so devastating. Any positive change makes us feel good and the brain remembers the feeling.

Dr. Gerald Edelman won a Nobel Prize for his work on the immune system and in his book *Neural Darwinism* argues that patterns of neural circuitry are not directed by external influences but by synapses in the brain that compete like animals in their environment to stay alive. Those synapses and neural routing maps that are used most often dominate "air time" and become easily recognized tunes. The more we can understand the hidden world of our own nature, the better we'll be at nurturing it and possibly prevent a lifetime of illness for ourselves or our children. You can be one of these people! It requires only proper intentionality to initiate a lifestyle of simple eating and living. There is really no alternative.

Alkalinity Enhances Mind-Body Circuitry

Your brain and body's circuitry are extremely sensitive to the slightest change in the pH level of your body's vital fluids. The pH scale runs from 1 to 14: a pH less than 7 is acidic; more than 7 is alkaline. Your body works hard to sustain several pH levels in various body systems. You want to maintain a balanced pH of 6.8 to 7.1 inside your cells. The most important pH is that of your blood, which is strictly controlled between 7.35 and 7.45 and is slightly alkaline. Your stomach fluid must be acidic, with a pH of 1.5 so it can digest food, but pancreatic fluid is very alkaline with a pH of 8.8. Your cerebrospinal fluid and brain require a balanced pH of 6.8 to 7.1.

Every day, your body produces organic, acidic by-products such as acetic acid, carbonic acid, fatty acids, lactic acid and uric acid, which it buffers or neutralizes with organic minerals from the vegetables, salads, herbs, spices, "green drinks" and fruit you eat. When your body's alkaline buffers are not eaten in sufficient daily quantities, toxic, acidic waste accumulates in the cells, causing enormous damage to your overall health. A comprehensive review comparing alkalinizing diets to acidic diets in the *American Journal of Clinical Nutrition* (no. 68, 1998) concludes that alkalinizing diets improve health, nitrogen balance, bone density and human growth hormone (hGH) concentrations. Acidic diets cause acidosis (low oxygen levels), bone loss (osteoporosis) and muscle mass loss. Acidosis appears to allow pathogens and cancer cells to proliferate, whereas an alkaline pH (high oxygen levels) discourages cancer cell colony initiation and promotion.

Acid-forming foods keep your central nervous system in a state of sympathetic dominance. This causes your adrenal glands to work overtime, which eventually depletes adrenal reserves and gives you that "drop-dead fatigue." Alkaline-forming foods promote a healthy state of parasympathetic dominance. This pH allows you to feel passionate about life and fully energized.

Measuring the pH of a food as it exists outside of the body is irrelevant. After a food is consumed, digested and absorbed, the final residue or "ash" is either alkaline, acidic or neutral depending on the mineral mix in the food. The minerals sulfur, phosphorus and iron form acid ions once inside the body. These minerals are found primarily in proteins, such as fish, poultry, meat, eggs, grains, legumes and most nuts and seeds. These foods are called acid-forming foods. Eating too many of these foods impose a net acidic overload on the body. The most acid-forming foods are the cola soft drink, coffee and alcohol, full of phosphoric and carbonic acids. If you consume too many of these foods your body will work hard to neutralize them with alkaline blood buffers, which then will not be available to neutralize other acidic products your body naturally produces as a by-product of cellular metabolism.

Sodium, potassium, calcium and magnesium form alkaline reactions once inside the body. These minerals are found primarily in fruits, salads, vegetables, herbs, spices and "green drinks," and are called alkaline-forming foods.

Note that not all acidic foods increase acidity inside your body. Lemon juice and apple cider vinegar are extremely acidic with a pH of 3.5 because of their citric acid content. However, in digestion the citric acid breaks apart, and the potassium and magnesium form alkaline ions called potassium or magnesium citrate, which actually increase alkalinity.

You need a daily 75 to 25 percent ratio of alkaline-forming and acid-forming foods, so try to consume approximately 75 percent of your foods from the alkaline-forming foods and 25 percent from the acid-forming foods. Metabolic acidosis (too acidic) or alkalemia (too alkaline) accelerates cellular, biological aging and prevents peak network neuropeptide and neurotransmitter communication. Keeping body fluids in acid/alkaline equilibrium is accomplished by (1) encouraging the neutralizing or buffering systems in the blood like sodium bicarbonate and potassium bicarbonate, (2) regulating the pH action of the lungs, and (3) regulating the pH action of the kidneys, which excrete more or less bicarbonate. Bicarbonate acts as an acid sponge in the body.

When you work or exercise hard you create an abundance of volatile liquid acids, so the depth and rate of your breathing automatically increase to remove carbonic acid by separating it into water and CO_2, exhaling CO_2 (carbon dioxide) through the lungs. Then the kidneys kick in by buffering excess acids in the urine with bicarbonates and expelling them.

Respiration—breathing deeply to oxygenate all of your deep tissues and 100 trillion cells—is the primary buffering system in the body. That is why I encourage you to daily take meaningful pauses and to deeply breathe in revitalizing, alkaline oxygen while removing stale, acidic carbon dioxide. Eating cell-friendly foods and deep breathing greatly aids the body's detoxification system and can keep your bones strong and your body cancer free.

A study in the 2003 journal *Neoplasma* details a study in which highly acidifying soft drinks, alcohol and coffee proved to be statistically significant risk factors for cancer. The *American Journal of Clinical Nutrition* presented research demonstrating that alkaline-forming foods build strong bones and prevent both risk of fracture and osteoporosis, while an excess of acidifying foods increase bone loss, risk of fracture and osteoporosis.

It is interesting to note that human cells are slightly alkaline and plant cells are slightly acidic. Plant cells leave an alkaline "ash" after being digested. If the human body remains in an acidic state for too long, human cells become acidic like plant cells, facilitating the initiation and promotion of cancer cell colonies.

Fruits are classified generally as alkaline due to the presence of citric, malic and succinic acids, which, after digestion, absorption and metabolism are converted into bicarbonate and water. Cranberries are an exception. Cranberries are rich sources of phenolic and benzoic acids that do not convert to bicarbonates but are excreted as acids. This is why cranberries are good for urinary infections.

The ability for foods to impact the acid-alkaline balance can be measured in your body through the Potential Renal Acid Load (PRAL) test.

The main message is to keep your body slightly alkaline by eating lots of colorful vegetables, salads, herbs, spices, "green drinks" and fresh fruit, which allows enzymes, hormones, neurotransmitters and neuropeptides to operate efficiently. (For a complete list of alkalinizing and acidifying foods, go to www.genuinehealth.com.)

You can incorporate dietary and lifestyle choices that boost and balance your alkalinity, good mood, vibrant energy, immune system, neurotransmitters and neuropeptides to experience your fulfilled and dynamic best self all life long. That's the purpose of this book: to help you make all those choices in the certainty that co-creating a life of vibrant vitality and dynamic well-being is about a process and commitment, not a destination.

Lifesaving Medicine Based on pH

Dr. Stephen Russell at the Mayo Clinic is a cancer specialist who knows how to use pH in a novel approach to seek, find and destroy cancer cells. The one characteristic of a malignant tumor is that it continues to divide extremely well with little or no oxygen in an acidic, anaerobic environment—the same acidic environment that bacteria and viruses need to replicate.

Using this knowledge, Dr. Russell and another cancer researcher, Dr. Kenneth Kinzler of Johns Hopkins Hospital's Kimmel Cancer Center, are rehabilitating bad bugs such as viruses and bacteria that operate well in an acidic, anaerobic environment into therapeutic lifesaving good bugs. Using the basic tools of molecular biology, Drs. Russell and Kinzler are redesigning with new instructions, and transforming common microbes like the clostridium, salmonella and c. botulinum bacteria or the Epstein-Barr virus (EBV) to attack a cancer cell, divide furiously, penetrate the malignant cell, continue to replicate, produce deadly natural toxins and destroy the cell from within. They have learned to attach molecular tracking proteins to the microbe to make sure that once it is set free, it does not deviate from its therapeutic mission of targeting cancer cells and spin out of control.

These are good microbes to use because if the microbe goes awry, the infection could be easily controlled with antibiotics or antiviral medications. Other microbiologists are modifying strains of viruses and bacteria to become ideal vehicles for delivering potent cancer drugs. Dr. Russell and Dr. Eva Galanis constructed a measles virus that recognizes and targets a mutation often found in brain tumor cells but never in normal cells.

More than 95 percent of the population is infected with EBV. Dr. Cliona Rooney, an immunovirologist at the Texas Medical Center, has retrained EBV to recognize, target and form identical protein bonds with three different types of cancer—throat cancer, Hodgkin's disease and non-Hodgkin's lymphoma. This cutting-edge idea is to have a therapeutically modified bacteria or virus exploit something unique to the cancer cell. The easiest method is to use rehabilitated, altered microbes like clostridium to replicate, like it also does, only in the oxygen-starved, acidic, anaerobic depths of a tumor. Once inside the cancer cell, the bacterium releases its toxins, which quickly eat through the malignant growth. This therapy has been tested only in mice, but with impressive results.

The bacterium salmonella and the measles virus have the ability to quickly zero in on tumor cells. In a small pilot study conducted at the Mary Crowley Medical Research Center in Dallas, two of three patients given the altered, rehabilitated salmonella had impressive results. These studies point to something more exciting.

Rehabilitating, retraining and re-outfitting bad bugs to be therapeutic, natural chemotherapy "good guys" attacking a malignant tumor at its acidic, anaerobic core is good mind-body medicine. The technology exists to make it an achievable goal.

Cellular biologists are learning to coat the sequestered, then altered, microbes with a protein coating that cloaks the microbe like a stealth bomber and renders it invisible to immune cell radar long enough so that they can deliver a lethal, natural "toxic drop" on a cancer cell's periphery—then eat into the acidic core of the cancer cell and destroy it. One thing is certain: medical research will undergo greater, more captivating changes during the next decade than in the last five hundred years to vastly expand both our mental and physical horizons. In the meantime, most researchers are keeping their pH slightly alkaline—and so should you.

This is the kind of high-impact change we can all benefit from.

18

IN PURSUIT OF HUMAN EXCELLENCE—BE HEALTHY... BE HAPPY!

Food that is healthy and food that gives pleasure are not mutually exclusive. I encourage people to upgrade their eating habits and lifestyle, to improve their energy, vitality, moods and well-being. For all people—from those struggling with mood, depression, sleep or energy problems, to those who just want to feel a little better—this book is a breath of fresh air. It promotes mental, physical, emotional and spiritual well-being over counting calories, measuring fat grams or calculating blocks of carbohydrates. *The Path to Phenomenal Health* provides an easy-to-follow blueprint for revitalizing and rejuvenating your brain and body. It helps you put your diet, mood, energy and lifestyle back on track, not just for the short term but for years to come.

We stand at a critical threshold, with the potential to enhance human intelligence and mind-body wellness—and expand our horizons. The rewards will be considerable.

Poor food choices send negative signals for flawed healing responses throughout your body and brain. Today we have to adapt wisely to our daily and moment-to-moment food selections, and to our busy daily lives, with a positive, calm-response lifestyle. Mae West once said, "You're never too old to become younger." I know for a fact that you're never too old to become younger *or* healthier.

ARE YOU OPERATING AT OPTIMUM PEAK PERFORMANCE LEVELS?

Our cells respond positively to healthy food prepared with love, care and attention, and negatively to food prepared artlessly and carelessly. If you eat healthy food, you should feel the satisfaction of being nourished, energized, happy and content.

The simplest cell-friendly meals can be extraordinarily satisfying if they are designed, prepared and served with the sole intention of nourishing, satisfying and rejuvenating. I begin all my meals with a thanksgiving and grace. I have trained myself to eat slowly and to savor my food.

Even the tiniest deficiencies could cause subtle and undetected disruption in peak mental and mind-body well-being. Roy Walford, MD, a world-renowned researcher who was at the University of California, Los Angeles Medical School, once told me, "Cognitive activity involves the coordinated activity of billions of neurons, countless biochemical pathways and many neuropeptides, and their associated neurotransmitters. It may well be that relatively small daily dietary deficiencies that are dismissed as causing only minor changes to the activity of a single neuron will, along with many other similar minor effects, have a measurable and potentially damaging cumulative influence on mind-body functioning and energy production."

> "I can't understand why people are frightened of new ideas. I'm frightened of the old ones."
>
> John Cage, author

Your brain and body may get enough vitamins, minerals, antioxidants, protein, water and nutrients to appear to function "normally," but are you operating at optimal peak performance? Many researchers, including myself, believe that substantial segments of the North American population may be nutrient deficient. Deterioration in physical, emotional and mental function previously attributed to "normal aging" may be due to undetected and correctable deficiencies in cell-friendly nutrients whose daily inadequate intake progressively accumulates, leading to excessive wear-and-tear far earlier in your life than you expect or want it to. You could be accelerating your very own aging process—far too soon!

It is now known that brain cells starving for critical micronutrients cannot function optimally, and wreak havoc on the delicate balance of brain chemicals. Kevin Worry, MD, of Victoria, British Columbia, said to me, "It's a new and powerful idea backed with adequate evidence to support the concept."

So much hard-core, scientific evidence substantiates the fact that modern North American society is riddled with a pernicious form of sub-clinical, symptomless, marginal malnutrition that most people have considered to be "normal." They endure lethargy, fluctuating weight, substandard moods, fragmented sleep, daytime fatigue and an undernourished brain and body for a lifetime. They are unaware that they have the immediate potential to be brighter, smarter and happier, with enormous energy, more enthusiasm and increased creativity—and feel better. Their current productivity at work and home can increase dramatically with a greater sense of satisfaction and fulfillment.

It seems incredible that each of us can reach for and achieve a more fulfilled, content, serene and happier life with optimum performance levels in our mental, physical, emotional and spiritual domains. I want you to attain this!

Can you be creatively adaptable to both your daily food and lifestyle choices? If you can, your immune system, brainpower, elevated mood and spiritual awareness will thank you by keeping you healthy, and your 100 trillion cells will dance with authentic joy; they will talk to you with a constant buzz of available energy, ready to respond to your daily needs. For example, your brain is saying you need to exercise, but if your body is saying "forget it," it's time to re-evaluate your lifestyle.

Energy is the currency of life. Energize yourself daily.

"When the power of love overcomes the love of power the world will know its peace."

Jimi Hendrix

IF YOU BUY PROCESSED FOODS, YOU'LL HAVE "BUYER'S REMORSE"

Unfortunately, the processed, degraded, prepackaged foods sold as convenience foods or fast foods may contain few, if any, nutrients. Saturated and trans fats "gum up" your intestines and create malabsorption mayhem and an energy crisis.

To add insult to injury, these foods are highly manufactured to look good, smell good and taste good, but they carry a deadly price tag. Full of sugar, sweeteners, trans fatty acids, salt, preservatives and taste enhancers to delight your taste buds, they are guaranteed to impair your physical, mental and emotional performance. The dilemma is that most of these refined foods are attractive because they are convenient and tasty, but contribute nothing at all to our vitality, creativity, brilliant brainpower and well-being. Brain cells slowly starve to death looking for nonexistent nutrients in processed food.

The time you save by eating at fast food restaurants is not worth the health complications it will cause. Please avoid exchanging convenience for your health and energy, which are far too precious to lose over a quick and inexpensive meal.

The prestigious British medical journal *Lancet* reported in 2005 on a study from Harvard Medical School that verifies the conclusions reached by Morgan Spurlock in his movie *Super Size Me*. Researchers found that eating fast food even two times a week could double your chances of developing insulin resistance, which often leads to full-blown diabetes, while packing on 15 extra pounds, leaving you de-energized. Those who had substandard nutrition were much more apt to be depressed, emotionally unstable, nervous, anxious, irritable, confused, uncertain, easily discouraged and fatigued.

Loren Cordain, MD, wrote a commentary in the February 2005 *American Journal of Clinical Nutrition*. His statement regarding refined or processed foods was: "Consequently, these foods negatively affect proximate nutritional factors, which underlie or worsen, virtually all chronic diseases of civilization."

Today a supermarket may contain 40,000 items, much of it processed foods made from refined grains, sugars, sweeteners and cheap fats, with annual North American sales of about US$210 billion. *Caveat emptor*, buyer beware is still the rule of thumb!

BY TWENTY-FOUR BRAIN DAMAGE BEGINS AND AT THIRTY-FOUR IT IS MEASURABLE—BUT IT IS REVERSIBLE!

I talked with Dr. Denham Harman, professor emeritus at the University of Nebraska, a Wise Elder still active in research into his eighties. He said, "The general health and longevity of our brain and body are initially shaped long before we are born by the antioxidants our mothers ingest before conception and during pregnancy."

Researcher Steven J. Schoenthaler at California State University says, "What is adequate to prevent physical signs and symptoms of malnutrition may not be adequate to prevent impaired mental function." Vincent DeMarco, MD, of Toronto says, "The genes are the bricks and mortar to build our brain, the environment through food choices and lifestyle is the architect."

Dr. Harman's early experiments show that pregnant mice given antioxidants had offspring that aged more slowly. Researchers have conclusively and overwhelmingly shown that animals fed cell-friendly foods, antioxidants and EPA- and DHA-rich fish oils stay healthier as they age; they suffer less degenerative disease, have far better mental ability and live longer. Dr. Harman feels that the earlier you start to care for your brain and body, the less they will deteriorate through the years and the more reliable they will be for you throughout your lifetime.

Age-related memory loss, dementia, Parkinson's disease, Alzheimer's, loss of brainpower and good moods do not begin when they are diagnosed. Loss of critical brainpower begins in preschoolers, continues in the teenage years if it is not repaired and escalates in our twenties, all the while remaining symptomless and insidious. The brain accumulates wear-and-tear from sugar, trans fats, stress, lack of exercise, sleep debt, insufficient antioxidants, inflammation and lack of EPA and DHA fish oil fats.

Dr. Harman points to an initial age between twenty-four to twenty-eight when antioxidant defenses have accumulated so much wear-and-tear that age-related damage begins eventually emerging as neurodegenerative brain damage with progressive loss of intelligence, memory, balance and fluid movement. By thirty-four years of age, almost everyone has easily measurable brain damage, called excitotoxic brain dysfunction, that progresses insidiously without symptoms.

As an example: "In many Alzheimer's patients, by their mid-30s, diseased neuronal cells, especially in the hippocampus, start to slowly fill with *black neurofibrillary tangles, tau and beta amyloid plaque* (protein clusters) that form gumlike blockage and choke brain cells to death," states Dr. Marianne Leblanc of Optima Health Solutions International in Vancouver, British Colombia.

Until recently, researchers felt that neurocellular gaps destroyed by Alzheimer's, Parkinson's, alcoholism, brain injuries, strokes and the aging process could never be reversed. Now, thanks to many visionary neuroresearchers, that old idea and scientific maxim has been proven wrong, leading to amazing new prospects of brain cell recovery, regrowth, expansion and rejuvenation at any age. Dr. Elizabeth Gould of Princeton University said, "It mandates new ways of thinking about the brain."

Note: Researchers at Columbia University in New York City studied 150 patients with mild cognitive impairment and compared their sense of smell to that of 63 healthy people between the age of forty-three to eighty-five at intervals of six months over a period of five years. The inability to smell strawberries, soap, menthol, clove, pineapple, lilac, natural gas and lemon was as good an indicator of the group's risk for Alzheimer's disease as were memory tests and fMRI scans. Furthermore, the *Archives of Neurology* highlighted clinical proof that daily use of the marine fatty acids "mood smart" EPA and "brain smart" DHA reduced the risk of Alzheimer's disease by 60 percent.

RUSTPROOF YOUR MIND AND BODY: A MODERN-DAY SOLUTION THAT WORKS

Denham Harman, MD, PhD, explains that throughout life all your cells, especially brain cells, are bombarded by thousands of attacks every day from unstable, heat-seeking chemical missiles called oxygen-free radicals. The energy system begins in your cells or, more specifically, in the tiny structures called mitochondria. It is interesting to note that 99 percent of our mitochondria are inherited from our mothers. Most cells contain from 500 to 3,000 mitochondria that can manufacture 150 pounds a day of the energy molecule adenosine triphosphate (ATP). The harder an organ works, the more energy it demands and makes.

The mitochondria in your brain are the hardest working. Unfortunately, approximately 5 percent of all the energy the mitochondria produce in your brain escapes like hot smoke from a factory, and produces a renegade free radical storm. This damage is inevitable and accumulates in everyone's brain and body. However, there are remarkable modern-day antioxidants that can do more than mop up collateral damage—they actually prevent any further damage. The beneficial antioxidant recipes that research recommends actually harness and de-energize free radicals before they cause inflammation and degenerative damage.

You want smart diversity in your strategic, global investment portfolio and likewise you want brilliant diversity in your daily, strategic antioxidant support for your body and brain. Renowned nutritional researcher Dr. Bruce Ames and colleagues at the University of California, Berkeley, have identified close to fifty genetic diseases, including cancer, that involve either defective vitamin-cofactor-binding sites or reactive oxygen species (ROS), free radicals reacting to oxygen that can be corrected by progressive use of therapeutic vitamin, mineral and antioxidant supplementation.

Here are two recipes for this antioxidant formula, to be taken with meals:

1. **If you are under fifty years of age, or even if you are beyond this age, and your memory, balance, mood, motivation and attention span are excellent, you can daily use:**

- 100 mg of R+, R-Dihydro or alpha lipoic acid (half at breakfast, half at supper)
- 1 serving of *greens+ extra energy* **or** *Life Extension Herbal Mix*
- 1,000 mg of acetyl-L-carnitine (half at breakfast, half at supper)
- 3 softgels, one at each meal, of enteric-coated wild fish oil concentrate, rich in "mood smart" EPA and "brain smart" DHA, and that also contain 400 mg of borage oil in each softgel for biologically active omega-6 essential fats
- 30–800 IU of vitamin E, which includes all eight forms of real vitamin E as alpha-, beta-, delta- and gamma-tocopherols plus alpha-, beta-, delta-, gamma-tocotrienols (half at breakfast, half at supper)
- 100 mg of Coenzyme Q10 (half at breakfast, half at supper) based on a blood test
- 3 capsules of an antioxidant formula, 1 at each meal, that contain vitamin A as mixed carotenoids, vitamin C as an ascorbate, selenium, n-acetyl-cysteine, lycopene, European bilberry, citrus bioflavonoids and full-spectrum grape extract
- 800 mg of turmeric (half at breakfast, half at supper)
- a food-based multivitamin mineral formula
- 6 macadamia nuts daily for the nearly forgotten omega-7 essential fats

2. If you are over fifty years of age or notice the telltale signs of memory loss, vision and hearing loss, a motivational downturn and loss of both attention span and good moods, you can daily use:

- 100 mg of R+, R-Dihydro or alpha lipoic acid (half at breakfast, half at supper)
- 1 serving of *greens+ extra energy* **or** *Life Extension Herbal Mix*
- 30–800 IU of Vitamin E, which includes all eight forms of real vitamin E as alpha-, beta-, delta- and gamma-tocopherols plus alpha-, beta-, delta-, gamma-tocotrienols (half at breakfast, half at supper)
- 250 mg of citicholine (cytidine diphosphate choline) at breakfast
- 1,000 mg of the amino acid L-carnosine (half at breakfast, half at supper)

- 300 mg of phosphatidylserine at breakfast
- 3 capsules of an antioxidant formula, 1 at each meal, that contain vitamin A as mixed carotenoids, vitamin C as an ascorbate, selenium, n-acetyl-cysteine, lycopene, European bilberry, citrus bioflavonoids and full-spectrum grape extract
- 1,000 mg of acetyl-L-carnitine (half at breakfast, half at supper)
- 1,000 micrograms (a high dose) of folic acid (half at breakfast, half at supper)
- 3 capsules, 1 at each meal, of enteric-coated wild fish oil concentrate, rich in "mood smart" EPA and "brain smart" DHA, that also contain 400 mg of borage oil in each softgel for biologically active omega-6 essential fats
- 100–400 mg of Coenzyme Q10 (half at breakfast, half at supper) based on a blood test
- 80 mg of resveratrol (half at breakfast, half at supper)
- 800 mg of turmeric (half at breakfast, half at supper)
- 400–1,000 IU of vitamin D3 (half at breakfast, half at supper)
- a food-based multivitamin mineral formula
- 10–50 mg sublingually of the combination of the hormones DHEA (dehydroepiandrosterone) and 7-kito DHEA, half before sleep, half before breakfast, and 1.5–5 mg of sublingual melatonin one hour before sleep (use pharmaceutical grade, natural, bio-identical hormones only under the supervision of a knowledgeable physician who understands *hormonerestorative therapy* and based on the results of your specific blood tests)
- 6 macademia nuts daily for the nearly forgotten omega-7 essential fats

Note 1: 7-kito DHEA (a metabolite of DHEA) does not convert to estrogen or testosterone but does boost immune function and helps to reduce body fat. Deficiencies of DHEA, after the age of forty, have been correlated with numerous age-related conditions such as cancer and heart disease. Your physician can easily test your blood to determine your DHEA status.

Note 2: Taking anticholesterol drugs not only lowers your cholesterol, but also tends to deplete your reserves of CoQ10 (coenzyme Q10), also known as ubiquinone, potentially leaving you with clean arteries but a dysfunctional brain. That's why if you are taking cholesterol-lowering drugs, called statins (prime examples are Lipitor, Mevacor and Zocor), you must be extra sure to take CoQ10 supplements to preserve your brain as well as your heart.

The National Institutes of Health estimates that by 2006, as many as 50 million North Americans could be using statin drugs to reduce cholesterol. These cholesterol-lowering drugs, technically called HMG-CoA reductase inhibitors, could possibly also inhibit critical CoQ10 biosynthesis in the liver. Your physician can quickly check your CoQ10 status with a blood test to determine if you require additional supplementation.

CoQ10 is a naturally occurring antioxidant that plays an important role in the synthesis of ATP (adenosine triphosphate), the universal energy currency of the body. CoQ10 helps with the regeneration and recycling of vitamins C and E and also helps with the metabolism (burning) of carbohydrates and fats. CoQ10 also plays an important role in protecting the body from various types of cancer and heart disease.

WE'RE NOT IN EDEN ANYMORE

The recommended daily intake of essential nutrients is intended to be available entirely through your food choices. In reality, it is impossible to get these nutrients through food because our commercial growing soils are depleted of many essential nutrients. The foods being grown today (except organically grown foods) have on average *30 to 50 percent lower quantities* of these essential antioxidants, phytonutrients, vitamins and minerals than they had in 1985.

Examine the results of just one research study. Ninety students were assigned to one of three groups. The first group received a multivitamin mineral supplement; the second group received an identical-looking placebo; and the third, nothing. After nine months, only the first group had a remarkable boost in their IQ—almost ten full points. An increase of just five points would allow almost 40 percent of ADD, ADHD and special needs students to graduate from special need classes and succeed in regular classes. Recently, a *New England Journal of Medicine* editorial stated, "The evidence suggests that people who take supplements, and their children, are healthier."

In the March 2005 issue of *Cancer Research*, Dr. Haojie Li, of Brigham and Women's Hospital in Boston, stated that "25 percent of men carry the AA variation of a specific gene called MnSOD which leaves them more susceptible to prostate cancer if their antioxidant levels are low." Previous research in women has linked a variation in the MnSOD gene with elevated risk for breast cancer in women who have low antioxidant status.

A study published in the March 2005 issue of the journal *Neurology* concludes that common dementia, memory loss and mild cognitive impairment, most often attributed to old age, are caused by undetected early Alzheimer's disease or reoccurring mini-strokes. The authors state, "the study shows that mild cognitive impairment is often the earliest clinical manifestation of two common age-related neurological diseases—Alzheimer's and vascular disease causing strokes." What to do? Each and every day, take these antioxidant formulas; keep your body and mind active; eat lots of alkalinizing, colorful vegetables, salads, fruits, herbs, spices, and energizing "green drinks"; reduce stress by meditating; and get deep sleep.

David A. Bennett, MD, the lead author of the study, states, "even mild loss of cognitive function in older people should not be viewed as normal, but as an indication of a disease process."

Better still, Dr. Richard Restak, a neuropsychiatrist at George Washington University Medical Center in Washington, D.C., emphasises that with proper care, damaged brain neurons can regain and reinstate some of that damage by (1) mobilizing the brain's inherent plasticity and (2) the communication networks in the brain recruiting additional healthy neurons, and allocating them to substitute and compensate for the damaged area.

The 2005 annual report of the American Cancer Society entitled *Cancer Prevention and Early Detection: Facts and Figures* estimates that healthier lifestyle practices and greater participation in cancer screening programs could immediately cut deaths from cancer by an enormous 50 percent.

Either way, these are the recipes for superior brainpower and peak performance for astonishing results for a lifetime. Even a minor delay will result in increased suffering. So if you have not been conscientious in caring for your brain and body before, then it is definitely a good time to start now.

Troublesome free radical renegades hit and tear at cell membranes, proteins and DNA at an estimated rate of one hundred thousand hits a day. This free radical storm causes the wear-and-tear you see in your skin, hair, robust vitality, memory and diminishing brainpower.

RENEGADE FREE RADICALS HIT AND TEAR AT CELLS

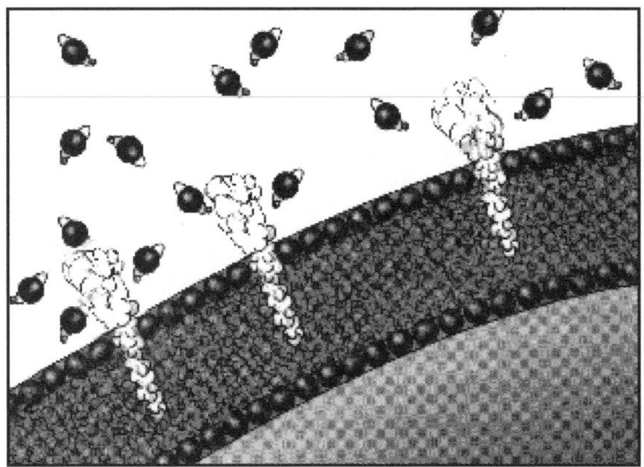

This damage begins showing up by age twenty-four, is measurable at thirty-four and continues to damage cells quietly, without any warning symptoms, and is cumulative, all life long. Antioxidants harness and de-energize free radicals.

YOUR LIFE IS NOT A SPECTATOR SPORT: DARE TO RESHAPE IT BETTER

You need to have great adaptability to survive, to take a successful, creative quantum leap, and to do what very few in western society before you have done—become a Wise Elder—and help all of humanity grow into a loving, compassionate, calmer, happier, healthier united family. We can do it one person at a time, beginning with ourselves—the power of one! On our journey to becoming Wise Elders, we can all become more energized and be ready to take on whatever learning challenges life may bring our way with emotional balance, spiritual maturity, love and gratitude. This is a radical departure from the accepted norm of growing older and fading away, forgotten in a nursing home. In 2004, the U.S. Centers for Disease Control in Atlanta reported that half of all North Americans living today will spend their latter years in nursing homes, unable to care for themselves. I don't want that for you!

Your future depends on all the choices you make each day. "Survival of the fittest" was a proper adaptation response for our ancient biological ancestors to survive and flourish. To survive and flourish well today, we must adapt by a new rule of the road: "survival of the wisest."

The prominent psychologist Abraham Maslow, who wrote *Motivation and Personality*, felt that we all function on a "hierarchy of needs." The pattern of our needs begins with survival requirements like food, shelter and safety. Once these basic needs are satisfied, we pursue meaning, love, self-esteem, social-esteem and, ultimately, the highest psychological need, self-actualization—the transformation of fully integrating all components of our mental, physical, emotional and spiritual personality, or self. Each level's needs must be at least partially met before those at the next level can motivate us to grow, change and transform.

> "The ability for change is phenomenal. That's what the brain does best: it adapts."
>
> Dr. Jay Giedd, psychiatrist, National Institutes of Health

The ancient mystery of how the brain works and how we can make it work even better is yielding to 21st century research and knowledge. The most advanced brain imagery technologies today are the functional magnetic resonance imaging (fMRI), the emerging single photon emission-computed tomography (SPECT) and the two-photon laser scanning microscopy (TPLSM). A given mental task, like remembering a name, may involve a complicated network of neurocircuits that interact in varying degrees with others throughout the brain—not like the parts in a machine, but like the diverse instruments in a symphony orchestra combining flutes, violins, piano, cymbals, drums, rhythm, resonance and volume to create a particular musical effect, mood or feeling.

WE ARE ALL HARDWIRED FOR SPIRITUAL MATURITY

Our goal is to guide our mental state away from self-destructive, restrictive emotions and toward a more content, compassionate and happier frame of being. Western neuroscientists, spurred on by the recent evidence of the brain's reshaping capability, have taken a keen interest in prayer and meditation. Can meditation change our brain?

Richard Davidson, PhD, and colleagues at the University of Wisconsin–Madison have been studying brain activity in Tibetan monks, both in meditative and in non-meditative states. Davidson and colleagues had shown in earlier studies that when people fall into negative emotions or temperaments, they displayed a pattern of persistent activity in regions of their right prefrontal cortex. In people with positive emotions or temperaments, the activity occurs instead in the left prefrontal cortex.

Davidson recently tested the prefrontal activity in volunteers from a high-tech company in Wisconsin. All the volunteers received flu shots, then were separated into two groups. One group of participants received eight weeks of meditation training, while the control group did not. At the conclusion of the study, the participants who had meditated daily showed a measurable and pronounced shift in brain activity from the right (moody, discontented) prefrontal cortex to the left (happier, contented) prefrontal cortex. Those who meditated also increased their antibodies from the flu shot by 50 percent more than those who did not meditate. Amazingly, the healthier immune response suggests that the meditation experience was a meaningful pursuit, and affected the body's health and well-being as well as the brain's state of happiness and purpose.

Prayer and meaningful pauses are lifestyle enhancers that offer the same promising results. Prayer and meditation involve significant and measurable physiological transformations. The time spent in these pursuits will reward you with a greater sense of well-being and optimism. Prayer and meditation offer an unprecedented opportunity to live life from an emotional and spiritual sense of abundance rather than scarcity. Their transforming qualities ignite a more positive attitude when exploring each day's challenges. Retake control of your life and experience the strong sense of your soul's contentment and fulfillment rather than pursuing more unfulfilled material pleasures and excitements.

So what else has recent research indicated?

Lesson 1: These scanning methods—fMRI, SPECT and TPLSM—do not provide a flurry of blips and flashes on a monitor but do provide extremely high-resolution images in 3D, like a hologram of individual dendritic spines and synapses in action for a quintillionth of a second. By using the fMRI, SPECT and TPLSM to get images of our brain, neuroscientists clearly show that meeting new challenges, changing, growing and transforming through both prayer and meditation enhance the growth, strength and performance of the left prefrontal cortex of the brain. This opens the brain's center of advanced learning, higher understanding, contentment, peace, equanimity and spiritual maturity.

"The ultimate question for each of us is namely, whether our brain's wiring created God, or whether God created our brain wiring," states neurotheologist Dr. Andrew Newburg. "In mystical experiences, both the content of the mind and sensory awareness drop out, so you are left with only consciousness," says Dr. Robert K.C. Formen, a scholar of comparative religion at Hunter College in New York City. He continues, "this tells you that consciousness does not need an object, and is not a mere by-product of sensory action."

Lesson 2: Recent research has found that the very active posterior superior parietal lobe of the brain—the orientation association area (OAA)—is the site that orientates us

> to physical reality, to time, to space, to a sense of individuality and separation from others and our physical surroundings. Prayer, meditation and meaningful pauses turn down the volume dial of the posterior superior parietal lobe's activity, as part of the brain's spiritual energy circuits, therefore allowing us to feel connected, "intimately interwoven with everyone and everything," as described by Dr. Newberg of the University of Pennsylvania, in his book *Why God Won't Go Away*. Once the OAA of our brain is turned down by calming alpha waves to about 8 Hz, we feel a sense of being limitless, non-local and in the *now*!
>
> During research in which their subjects were people who had been meditating and praying for many years, Newberg and his associates captured brain images of people in the midst of spiritual experiences. The pictures showed that the mind-body connection to genuine spiritual maturity is real. Daily, we need to supply the exact nutrients to support superior neuronal revitalization, receptor sensitivity, and high-fidelity performance of the neuropeptides and neurotransmitters.

Meeting and learning from life's daily challenges, prayer, meditation and meaningful pauses are no longer optional—they are mandatory. To allow our brains to reconstruct, revitalize, grow and transform for a lifetime, we must incorporate these life-enhancing strategies into each and every day. Globally, researchers now agree that after reaching maturity, the human brain, for better or for worse, is constantly changing and reshaping itself in response to stress, hormones, neurotransmitters, neuropeptides, diet and lifestyle choices. Dr. Michael Merzenich of the University of California, San Francisco, a pioneer in understanding brain plasticity, says, "what we now appreciate is that the brain is continually revising itself throughout life."

Neuroscientists agree that even if some neurons in your brain become non-operational because of abuse or disease, if you engage in an aggressive, supplemental antioxidant program, along with proper diet and lifestyle changes, new nerve connections can reach out across the brain to occupy neural real estate that had been left vacant for future development. This is the kind of brain we need for "survival of the wisest"!

NANOTECHNOLOGICAL ADVANCES

Technology has been snowballing, accelerating exponentially since the dawn of our species, slowly leading to radical shifts in the socio-economical framework of society. As a discovery is made, the doors to other mysteries open, which in turn open more doors in a cascade of advancement. It literally took eons for language to evolve, millennia to master writing, centuries for the development of the printing press and Morse code, decades to lead to the computer age, and in only a few short years the Internet has gone from nonexistent to universally pervasive.

Computer researchers predict that by 2015, a $1,500 computer will have the processing power of a human brain. By 2030, a $1,500 computer will have the processing power of two hundred human brains. By 2050, the exponential achievements will allow $1,500 to buy the processing power of ten thousand human brains. For example, the neuronal connections in our brains compute at two hundred transactions per second, which is millions of times slower than today's microchip electronic circuits.

NANOTECHNOLOGY AND YOU

Nanotechnology allows machines to be constructed at the atomic level. These nanomachines and nanobots will be able to monitor moods or individual atoms like neurotransmitters, neuropeptides and peptides do now, but with far greater consistency, precision and benefit.

"Nanotechnology" is a term invented by K. Eric Drexler in the 1970s to describe the study of objects whose smallest features are less than 100 nanometers (a nanometer is a billionth of a meter). Nanotechnology theorists believe these machines will not just make voyages of pure discovery, but will most often be sent on missions of cellular inspection, repair and reconstruction.

- There are various labs presently learning ways to create bloodstream-based biological microelectromechanical systems (bioMEMS) that intelligently seek and find pathogens and deliver precise medication. Kazushi Ishiyama, PhD, at Tohoku University in Japan, has developed micromachines that use microscopic spinning screws to deliver drugs directly into small cancerous tumors.
- Microelectronic mechanical systems (MEMS) are creating microscopic hydrogen fuel cells to power nanobots to help nanoengineered bloodstream-based devices to deliver hormones like dopamine precisely to the neurons of Parkinson's patients.
- Nanosurgery will use nanobots to destroy cancerous tumors cell by cell, or clear arteries of clogging plaque or perform surgery inside a cell, such as repairing and reconstructing DNA within the nucleus.
- Boston University's Timothy Gardner has developed a cellular logic switch, capable of turning nanobots into computers.
- Most degenerative diseases like cancer, cardiovascular disease, Alzheimer's, and type II diabetes are the result of the interaction between genetic and environmental factors. New testing for genetic factors, called genomics testing panels, are now available. As our DNA molecules replicate to create all the cells and tissues in the body, they can experience an alteration. These alterations are called polymorphisms (the state of assuming many shapes). The most common variety is single-nucleotide polymorphisms called SNPs (pronounced snips). Each person has approximately one million SNPs. Predictive genomics attempts to identify the most significant SNPs to determine how likely you are to be predisposed to develop a specific illness or disease, like cancer, cardiovascular disease or diabetes. Different ethnic groups have distinct SNPs. Genomic testing is now available for many SNPs to determine what genetic mutations you may have.

Today you can also find out through genomics testing what SNPs you have and modify the expression of genes you were born with through a cell-friendly diet, knowledge, therapeutic supplements and lifestyle choices. For a nanomedicine physician near your go to www.nanomedacademy.org.

REWRITE YOUR BODY'S OWNER'S MANUAL

Shangri-La: Today's Mystery Will Be Tomorrow's Awareness

Shangri-La can be here and now. Our own conscious awareness can set us all free from self-imposed doubt, pain, fear, anxiety and limitation. Be happy and you'll make others happy, too. Why would you deprive the world of all you have to offer life and—more significantly—deprive yourself of all the challenges and transforming growth the world has to offer you? "Long before we become ill, our body sends strong signals that something is wrong," states Dr. Joey Shulman. Before you feel the first chest pain of heart disease, find yourself challenged by cancer, become forgetful or need a hip replacement, the 100 trillion cells in your body and mind cry out daily for help and intervention. The potential in terms of enhancing and restoring human health and well-being is nothing short of spectacular. We human beings have a great deal more power to control our own destinies than we ever imagined. You can witness an astounding revitalizing and rejuvenating transformation in yourself.

> "She had made the best of time and time returned the compliment."
> Joseph Campbell, creative thinker

The old approach has been to deal with and tackle one ailment at a time—unfortunately, after the fact! Like a stack of dominoes or a house of cards, one by one, each system topples. "Aging is not a single 'quick fix' linear progression, but a group of inter-related biological processes," states Carolyn DeMarco, MD. However, for the first time in the experience of our human species, medical science, backed by accumulating evidence, suggests that illness, disease and dementia are not an inevitable part of life, nor necessarily a consequence of growing older. How long does your car last? The answer obviously depends on how well you take care of it.

Be grateful you are alive. Learning, growing and transforming today accomplishes half the job. To better handle tomorrow's challenges and to handle well the next day's, and the next's, and the next's is our full-time job. We must transform and become wiser and healthier every single day for a lifetime. This is the ultimate example of the power of emotional self-perpetuation.

Most of the time, our physical, emotional, mental and spiritual balance is maintained automatically, but there are many days when we must rebalance ourselves. Balance is wellness, and to be unbalanced is to be unwell. In nature, all living systems and energy fields maintain themselves through a continuous give and take, expansion and contraction. Foods, moods and lifestyle choices do just that. They expand or contract our energy and emotions; they acidify or alkalinize us. The pendulum swing of our cellular metabolism between those opposites is what keeps us more or less stable. If the pendulum stays too long on one side, our physical, mental, emotional or spiritual balance is disrupted and we feel unwell. Stay balanced—it is as simple as that.

Pursuit of human excellence in just one of our energy centers, whether mental, physical, emotional or spiritual, is not sufficient. Excellence in one of these energy regulators is not a fix or an antidote for poor performance in any other area. All of our energy centers must work *synergistically*. The total benefits gained by applying positive change and transformation in all four centers are exponentially greater than the benefits of any one alone.

> "If I had known I would live so long, I would have taken better care of myself."
>
> George Burns, on his 100th birthday

You must take advantage of the learning potential from everyday challenges. No matter what dilemmas or quandaries we face—health crises, relationship issues, financial stress, social challenges, emotional turmoil, anger, rage, cynicism, disappointment, natural catastrophes and global challenges of our time—we can always pursue and find a noble idea. We can implement this noble idea, and we, as the blessed human species, can prevail with love, optimism, hope, motivation, patience and endless effort. Amazingly, we can work with and overcome these necessary life challenges for a civilization-wide, worthwhile and achievable goal—the remarkable pursuit of human excellence.

George Bernard Shaw stated it nicely when he said, "We don't stop playing because we grow old, we grow old because we stop playing."

We can see a glimmer of light in darkness and a ray of hope in hopelessness.

Keep Your Mind-Body Connection Balanced

Mounting evidence clearly indicates that our moods can be the first indicators that we are out of balance. Psychosomatic illness, a long-accepted category of modern medicine and psychology, is one in which bodily dysfunction is caused by mental or emotional conditions like stress, anxiety, depression, insomnia, loneliness and staleness, with no meaningful direction in our life.

But the reverse is equally true. Our bodies' conditions affect our mental or emotional states with similar intensity. For example, hunger can cause moodiness, an energy crisis and aggression; a lack of sleep causes poor memory; and a lack of EPA omega-3 essential fats causes depression. Blushing, laughing or crying are all physical reactions caused by mental or emotional states. A recent study at the Mayo Clinic proved that type II (adult onset) diabetics were 66 percent more apt to develop all types of dementia, and had more than twice the risk of developing Alzheimer's disease. Diabetics were 300 percent more apt to develop dementia and Alzheimer's in a recent large-scale study at the University of California at Davis. However, the early stages of dementia in diabetics are preventable or reversible if diabetics follow the regimen recommended in this book. **Main message**: compromising your physical health over long periods of time is outright dangerous for your body and can be detrimental to optimal brain function for a lifetime.

Mountains of stunning evidence have piled up in the last few years documenting the mind-body connection as real, eminent and powerful. Neuroscientists have mapped pathways linking mental states to physical ones and vice versa. Our modern-day "survival of the wisest" challenge is to learn how to navigate them wisely, at will. Kenneth Pelletier, MD, clinical professor of medicine at the University of Arizona and the University of Maryland medical schools, states, "We want to know why so many people still aren't using mind-body medicine, when research has shown it to be strikingly effective for an enormous number of conditions."

Expand Your Human Potential—Get a Myers' Cocktail Tune-Up

Whether you are driven by intellectual curiosity or concern for your own personal wellness, consider the awesome benefits to human health and longevity promised by the leading edge of medical science—and what you can do today to take full advantage of these life-enhancing advances. The present state of our collective knowledge in the diverse fields of biology, medicine, miniaturization, and information technology is a bridge to a healthy future for those who dare to navigate the journey from ordinary to remarkable in twenty-one days.

If you do not feel well, you may choose to be progressive and seek out a physician who does intravenous micronutrient therapy (IVMT), which is sometimes referred to as the "Myers' cocktail." The late John Myers, a Baltimore physician, pioneered the therapy in the 1970s as a treatment for fatigue, depression, fibromyalgia, memory loss, poor skin tone, insomnia and even chest pains. After his death in 1984, Alan Gaby, another Baltimore physician, began to administer his own version of the cocktail, which is an intravenous infusion of a high-dose combination of superabsorbable vitamins, minerals, antioxidants and phytonutrients based on your personal biological needs as determined by blood tests. The IV administration is painless and takes only 15 minutes. The nutrients go directly into your bloodstream without having to go through the gastrointestinal tract. The immediate infusion of micronutrients strengthen the immune system, improve cellular membrane quality, boost cellular energy production and help blood vessels dilate more effectively, enhancing blood flow and dynamic energy to your 100 trillion cells.

"By 2015, if you stay healthy, emotionally balanced, and have an open mind, nanotechnology will usher in promising new approaches that will enable you to greatly improve your mind-body well-being by integrating your biological systems with new human-created technologies," states Daniel F. Leavitt, MD, of Salt Spring Island, British Columbia. Something that those before you could only dream of!

CHALLENGE, COMMITMENT, CURIOSITY AND CREATIVITY

You may see change as a challenge, or you may see challenge as an opportunity to change. Either way, you must use your commitment, curiosity and creativity to bring about a positive result for human growth from an otherwise difficult situation. A challenge is what life gives us many times a day. While sometimes difficult, challenges are worthwhile and meaningful for each of us. Commitment is the ability to put a priority on working with the challenge, knowing it is only an opportunity for growth toward human excellence and not a sacrifice. Curiosity is a desire to improve our health, knowledge, emotional balance and spirituality and to discover new wonders. We can benefit from improving the balance of our mind-body connection and—our human blessing—the ability to cope and learn from life's challenges.

Breathtakingly simple, wouldn't you agree? And getting there is easy!

"The universe is full of magical things, patiently waiting for our wit to grow sharper."

Eden Phillpotts, author

PURSUE HUMAN EXCELLENCE

Be the Solution—Imagine That!

Protect your faithful, hard-working cells. Give your 100 trillion cells natural, cell-friendly foods, water, balanced emotions and positive lifestyle choices so they can have the highest quality fuel possible. The assembly line of your cells will then be able to give you a lifetime of enormous energy, great moods, brainpower, spiritual maturity and an awesome overall feeling of well-being. Remember, your dynamic brain's circuitry and cell signalling systems enlarge and become more efficient with daily new challenges and cell-friendly foods as nutritional therapy.

THE SCIENCE BEHIND "AN APPLE A DAY"

Quercetin is a major dietery polyphenol present in high concentrations in apples, especially pigments in apple skins, onions and green tea. German researchers recently discovered that quercetin helps prevent colon cancer because it turns off various proteins involved in the growth of colon cancer cell colonies. Quercetin is a powerful antimutagenic compound to keep handy in your genetic toolbox.

These simple lifestyle suggestions are easy-to-implement actions that re-program your biochemistry to favorably change the ancient programs in your genes. This is a brave new approach to promote a better cycle of life for your lifetime experience. Be perpetually optimistic. Laugh and the joy will course through your 100 trillion delighted cells, boosting your immune system, rewiring and reshaping your brain, giving you a larger memory board. This joy will ripple throughout all humankind.

Dr. Robert Vogel and colleagues at the University of Maryland Medical Center measured test subjects' arteries before and after they sat and watched funny movies like *Mrs. Doubtfire, Snow Dogs* and *Kingpin*. After the subjects laughed, chuckled, cackled and howled for 60 minutes, their arteries expanded by an average of 22 percent, allowing blood, oxygen and fuel to reach more cells without as much strain. What was the conclusion? Just 1 hour of laughter is equivalent to the cardiovascular benefits of 30 minutes of jogging.

When we laugh and smile, the stress hormone levels of cortisol and adrenaline decline by 70 percent and our "feel good" hormone DHEA, the neurotransmitters dopamine and serotonin and the neuropeptide beta-endorphin levels soar by 40 percent. This is a simple but effective survival technique to give yourself a "home-court advantage"!

Why laugh and smile? Telomeres are DNA sequences or "tails" on DNA that get shorter every day when a cell divides, literally limiting our lifespan. Longer telomeres are associated with a younger biological age and a longer lifespan. *New Scientist* reports that researchers at the University of California discovered that stress does shorten telomeres. High stress, as elevated cortisol levels, shortened telomeres, thus accelerating our cellular age by 10 to 17 years. The shorter the telomeres, the shorter the cells' lifespan and the faster the body deteriorates. As more cells die, the effects of aging kick in: muscles weaken, memory slips, skin wrinkles, hair lacks lustre and motivation declines. Suddenly at 30 years of age we look and feel 45; at 40 we look and feel 55; at 50 we look and feel 65 and at 70 we look and feel 85. This is called accelerated aging.

Chronological age is your age on your driver's license or birth certificate. Biological age, which we can decelerate, is the age of your cells, glands, organs and immune systems. Our goal is to maintain a healthy and robust biological age that is 10 to 15 years younger than our chronological age. What does this mean? This means that with a wise and well-balanced lifestyle, a 40-year-old person using his or her genetic toolbox to follow the recommendations in this book could be physiologically and biologically operating equivalent to a super healthy 25-year-old. Likewise, a 60-year-old person could be operating at peak performance—disease free, robust, energetic, with great brainpower equivalent to a healthy 45-year-old. Amazingly, at 80 years of age you could live an enhanced life equivalent to a vibrant 65-year-old and at 100 years of age, that of a dynamic 85-year-old. "It is not a matter of looking 20 when you're 55, but looking good, vibrant and healthy for your age," states physician extraordinaire Zoltan Rona, MD, of Toronto.

Robert Keith Wallace, an American physiologist, measured the influence that meditation has on biological age. He discovered that meditators who had meditated for 5 years or more were *12 to 15* years biologically younger than their chronological age.

If happiness is the immune system's booster, then guilt and regret are its nemesis. Guilt and regret serve to modify behavior that we consider unacceptable by initiating mental punishment as our sentence. Excessive guilt and regret lead to depression and suppress our immune system. A Wise Elder, or one in training to be, would live each day mindful of his or her thoughts, words and actions, thus limiting guilt or regret. You can apply this strategy, starting today.

The Benefits of Voluntary Calorie Restriction

In 1986, when Leonard Guarente, PhD, proposed to study the biology of aging via calorie restriction (CR), his colleagues laughed at the proposition and called it bio-babble. What he found is that calorie restriction can increase lifespan for most animals and mammals. Roy Walford, MD, of UCLA, made great strides in understanding CR and why a drop in excess calorie intake could activate the gene SIR2 in yeast and SIRT1 in humans to help prolong life. Leonard Guarente and colleagues from the University of Wisconsin and from Johns Hopkins, and Dr. David Sinclair of Harvard are at the head of the research class today and focus on sirtuins, the family of proteins produced by SIR2 or its human analogue, SIRT1. They have found that a daily diet high in nutrients but low in calories (absolutely no junk food) magnifies the effects of sirtuins. Yeast with more sirtuin levels live longer. Mice that consume 30 percent fewer calories than what the average mouse eats have higher sirtuin levels and live an incredible 50 percent longer, virtually disease free.

David Sinclair's work has been focused on resveratrol (the polyphenol prominent in grapes, especially dry red wine), and with large doses, he increases SIR2 and prolongs lifespan in yeast by 70 percent.

Calorie restriction is an extremely effective strategy for survival during famines when it's imperative, not a choice. The SIRT1 gene kicks in to slow down aging, and pitches in to produce extra energy during a famine. All animals, including humans, can do this. It now appears that each species has an actual fixed number of calories that it can burn in a lifetime. By eating fewer calories each day and choosing highly nutritious foods, there will be more days left in your life until the calorie count is exhausted. All human cells are heat- and energy-producing engines. Cellular engines wear out from the amount of fuel or calories they consume, not from their chronological age. When you eat high-nutrient, low-calorie, cell-friendly foods each day, your remaining life expectancy will move steadily into the future. When you eat fewer calories but more nutrients, your SIRT1 gene kicks in to prolong your lifespan and, in the process, gives you an energy boost, which is good mind-body medicine.

What can you do to reap these results? Eat a minimum of eleven calories a day per pound of your ideal weight if you want to lose weight, twelve calories a day per pound of your weight if you want to maintain your weight and thirteen calories a day per pound of your ideal weight if you want to gain weight. For example, a woman with an ideal weight of 130 pounds should consume 130 × 12 = 1,560 calories daily to maintain her weight and a man of 165 pounds would require 165 × 12 = 1,880 calories a day to maintain his weight. Follow the dietary recommendations in this book so you will fuel up on satisfying and healthful foods high in nutrients and low in calories. The more excess calories we eat daily, the more heat and destructive free radicals we produce, thus accelerating our cellular engines' accumulated wear-and-tear. The quickest way to accelerate your biological age is unrestricted eating. Less is really proving to be more!

DARE TO NAVIGATE THE JOURNEY FROM ORDINARY TO REMARKABLE

The Path to Phenomenal Health is a journey into the emerging future.

My dietary and lifestyle modifications may seem, at first, like a lot to try and incorporate into your life. But if you are willing to give it a chance—just one day at a time—you'll find an authentic, whole new world of robust vitality, emotional balance and remarkable brainpower awaiting you. Do not deprive yourself or others of all that you can be. Take the journey and follow the path toward ever greater mind-body well-being.

These manageable steps and actions show you how to embrace food as "energy"—not as the "enemy" and, better yet, how to understand that eating is a pleasure instead of an emotional battle. Cell-friendly foods will contribute to your well-being and enhance your vitality based on your particular biological needs.

I cannot emphasize enough that you must commit yourself to your own well-being. Be proactively involved in daily shaping and reshaping the story of your life. Most intriguingly, you can promote the birth of actual new brain cells—an idea that was globally regarded as preposterous until recently. You can forestall and eliminate most chronic diseases. Staying balanced and energized each day will always be a "present time" challenge.

Re-Evaluate and Upgrade Your Personal Appraisal

Our biological ancestors evolved in an era of scarcity—environmental and biological choices described and defined them. Today we live in an era of increasing abundance—lifestyle and knowledgeable choices describe and define us. Improper food, knowledge and lifestyle choices underlie our modern-day epidemic of age-related degenerative diseases. Even the most minor biochemical failures accumulate daily and lessen your peak performance for a lifetime.

My philosophy is to provide you with optimal recommendations based on the latest persuasive, consistent and effective research. Pursue human excellence, not human perfection. Do it one day at a time. This is the secret to a much better, happier and more fulfilling life, forever. That is all I ask of you. Remember, one great day *equals* one great life. Challenge yourself to explore your dynamic potential and have fun while you do it. The evidence, I think, compels all of us to look at our own mind-body connection with new respect and optimism, knowing that its well-being and destiny are truly up to each of us. It is never too early or too late to decide to shape and re-shape your own life's destiny.

The human species is unique in seeking to expand its horizons and to reach beyond current limitations of our biological machinery. We are also the only species that can change our interpretation, perspective, perception, expectation and motivation and actually create or discover knowledge or imagine a desired emerging result such as transforming ourselves so we will become fulfilled, peaceful, happy and content. No noble idea, solution or creative quantum leap in human consciousness or awareness can ever happen in the physical world of matter—it can happen in sheer wonder only in the deep recesses of the blessed human mind and creative imagination.

All revolutions usually begin with an individual. The peak performance and wellness revolution is no different. It all comes down to "the power of one."

Q: Sam, how often is enhancing people's well-being on your mind?

A: All the time—with optimism and passion.

Literally and metaphorically, we have all come a long way. We all have peak performance within our immediate grasp. The possibilities are endlessly seductive if we can just muster the courage and willpower. That's the real hope. This can be an amazing time in your life.

Your decisions have implications for all those lives you are privileged to touch. All personal triumphs begin with tasks that seemed too difficult and incredibly daunting—but that shouldn't scare us.

Today, nanomedicine research and mind-body medicine can light the emerging pathway to our own optimal well-being. Walking it is still up to us!

I am asking you to tread carefully, and stop imprisoning yourself in restrictive, self-limiting concepts and a "stale habit syndrome" that diminish you. Instead, you should enhance your fundamental freedom of choice. Give yourself an unconditional pardon and initiate an amazing transformation in yourself and the way you live every day that will continue for many more years after this last page is read. A whole new world of possibilities opens to those who dare to transform themselves. You can be among them!

Become an enlightened Wise Elder, and maybe more!
Seek personal and global well-being in your lifetime.

"If wrinkles must be written upon our brows, let them not be written upon the heart. Your spirit should never grow old."
John Kenneth Galbraith

Now embark on a new journey—into life!

MEDICAL RESOURCES

There are many outstanding medical clinics in North America that will help you master this book and dramatically boost your wellness, brainpower and robust vitality. I will mention an example of one in Canada and one in the United States staffed by knowledgeable health practitioners. Please go to www.genuinehealth.com for a detailed list of cutting-edge clinics in your area.

Optima Health Solutions International
828 West 8th Avenue
Vancouver, B.C. V5Z 1E2

Phone: (604) 266-5338 or toll free (866) 878-0116
Fax: (604) 267-0911
Website: www.optimahealthsolutions.com

Medical Staff: Dr. Aslam Khan, DC, founder and director
Dr. Marianne Leblanc, MD, medical director
Dr. Nasif I. Yasin, MB, pain specialist

This is an impressive medical clinic specializing in revolutionary medical, chiropractic and prolotherapy (pain control) protocols. The clinic offers complete hormone, vitamin, mineral and antioxidant blood testing—total realignment of the body—and the most advanced pain-control protocols.

Note: Dr. Aslam Khan is remarkably dedicated, knowledgeable and far ahead of his time with unique, non-invasive approaches called the Khan Kinetic Therapy. I personally experienced a bad fall of 15 feet, landing on the back of my neck and head, upside down. I lost my vision, hearing and speech. Dr. Khan's work with me was remarkable, restoring my neurological circuitry.

Dr. Marianne Leblanc is at the leading-edge of advanced medical practices and is an expert in the field of antiaging medicine and bio-identical hormone replacement therapy.

Dr. Nasif Yasin specializes in advanced pain control using a glucose-based compound he injects directly to the area of injury, inflammation, arthritis, tendonitis or ligament and cartilage micro-tears. I believe this protocol, called prolotherapy, is the best pain relief approach available. Dr. Yasin is a pain control master who dramatically helped me with two serious sports-related injuries.

The PATH Medical Services and Research Foundation
185 Madison Avenue
New York City, NY 10016

Phone: (212) 213-6155
Fax: (212) 213-6188
Website: www.pathmed.com

Medical Staff: Dr. Eric R. Braverman, MD, director

Eric R. Braverman, MD, is brilliant and utilizes both conventional and alternative protocols in tandem. By merging internal medicine and neuropsychology, this new form of mind-body medical care treats your brain, your mind and your body as one entity. Dr. Braverman is able to deal with health issues that are the result of imbalances in your brain biochemicals.

Note: Please look at Life Extension Foundation www.lef.org to determine what hormonal blood tests you may need to determine your hormone status, and the ideal bloodstream range to be in for your age.

PRODUCT RESOURCES

ENERGIZING, ALKALINE, FOOD-BASED "GREEN DRINKS"

Not all concentrated "green drinks" are of the same high quality. *greens+* is the only multi-award-winning, clinically proven "green drink" formula tested by the University of Toronto Medical School and School of Pharmacology that proved to boost energy, antioxidant levels, alkalinity and increase well-being. It has won a gold medal on many occasions in both Canada and the United States from the Canadian Health Food Association and National Nutritional Foods Association as "Product of the Year," and The Inventors Club of America, Inc.'s prestigious International Hall of Fame award for exceptional quality.

In Canada
greens+
greens+ extra energy
greens+ kids
greens+ multi+
greens+ daily detox
are available from:

Genuine Health
Toronto, Ontario
Toll-free: (877) 500-7888
Website: www.genuinehealth.com

In the United States
greens+ is available from:

Orange Peel Enterprises, Inc.
Vero Beach, Florida
Toll-free: (800) 643-1210
Website: www.greensplus.com

Life Extension Herbal Mix is available from:
Life Extension
Ft. Lauderdale, Florida
Toll-free: (800) 544-4440
Website: www.lef.org

LONG-CHAIN OMEGA-3 ESSENTIAL FATTY ACID FISH OILS RICH IN "MOOD SMART" EPA AND "BRAIN SMART" DHA

Following the brilliant research of omega-3 fatty acid researchers such as Dr. Artemis P. Simopoulos, president of The Center for Genetics, Dr. Joseph Hibbelin of the National Institutes of Health,

Dr. Zanarini of Harvard Medical School, Dr. Bruce J. Holub of the University of Guelph and Dr. Alan Logan, director of CAM Research Consulting in New York, Genuine Health in Canada and the United States has formulated and developed id System enteric-coated wild, triple fish oil formulations to therapeutically help with specific conditions. These pharmaceutical-grade fish oils are either steamed or molecularly distilled.

Recent research highly recommends that you daily consume 650–1,000 mg of EPA and DHA for general use. For depression, 1,500 mg of EPA is routinely used on a daily basis. For heart health, you need a minimum of 300 mg of EPA, 200 mg of DHA and 1,200 mg of omega-6 borage oil. For a remarkable boost in supercritical brainpower, consider 300 mg of EPA and 750 mg of DHA daily.

North Americans consume only 130 mg of combined EPA and DHA per day—at least 520 mg short of the minimum 650 mg recommended by essential fatty acid experts worldwide.Adolescents between the age of eleven to seventeen go through a second stage of tremendous brain growth and can increase their intelligence, skin quality and good mood with "mood smart" EPA and "brain smart" DHA rich fish oil concentrates.

In Canada and the United States
Genuine Health Toronto, Ontario Toll-free: (887) 500-7888
Website: wwwgenuinehealth.com

1. *o3mega*: 180 mg EPA and 120 mg DHA per softgel for general use

2. *o3mega extra strength*: 400 mg EPA and 200 mg DHA for maximum benefits of o3mega

3. *o3mega+ pump*: 105 mg EPA, 69 mg DHA and 400 mg borage oil per softgel for a healthy cardiovascular system, provides the exact 4:2 ratio of EPA/DHA:GLA

4. *o3mega+ fit*: 146 mg EPA, 96 mg DHA and 225 mg borage oil per softgel for those exercising or on a diet because both lose EPA and DHA reserves quickly

5. *o3mega+ think*: 100 mg EPA and 250 mg DHA per softgel for a bright, alert boost in brainpower, cognitive function and maintenance of your eyes and nerves

6. *o3mega+ joy*: 500 mg EPA and 25 mg DHA per softgel for enhanced, superior, improved mood and well-being; scientific studies prove EPA regulates depression

BORAGE OIL, BLACK CURRANT OIL

In Canada
Omega Nutrition Canada Inc.
Toll-free: (800) 661-3529
Website: www.omegaflo.com

In the United States
Omega Nutrition U.S.A. Inc.
Toll-free: (800) 661-3529
Website: www.omegaflo.com

ENRICHED FLAX OIL WITH LIGNANS

In Canada and the United States
Spectrum Organic Enriched Flax Oil with 8 percent flax seed lignans
Spectrum Organic Products Inc.
Website: www.spectrumorganics.com

EVENING PRIMROSE OIL

In Canada and the United States
Efamol
Toll-free: (888) 318-5222
Website: www.efamol.com

HEMP SEEDS, PROTEIN AND OIL

In Canada and the United States
Manitoba Harvest
Toll-free: (800) 665-4367
Website: www.manitobaharvest.com

Bioriginal Food Corp.
Phone: (306) 975-9268
Website: www.intro@freshhempfoods.com

HIGH ALPHA WHEY ISOLATE PROTEIN POWDER—*proteins+*

In Canada and the United States

Genuine Health
Toll-free: (877) 500-7888
Website: www.genuinehealth.com

SUGGESTED SUPPLEMENTS

In Canada and the United States

- *abs+*; CLA and green tea EGCG have been proven in clinical trials to enhance significant abdominal fat reduction and weight loss, safely and naturally: www.genuinehealth.com
- Life Extension *Herbal Mix*, pharmaceutical grade CoQ10, resveratrol, DHEA, sublingual melatonin, vitamin E as tocopherols and tocotrienols: www.lef.org
- Turmeric 400 mg (11 percent curcumins–35.2 mg)—New Chapter Inc.: www.newchapter.info
- Super-absorbable CoQ10—HVL Inc.: www.Qmelt.com, and Twin Labs: www.twinlabs.com
- *pure calm de-stress kit*, soothes frazzled nerves—"Zen in a bottle": www.genuinehealth.com
- *greens+multi+*—award-winning food-based multi-vitamin/mineral: www.genuinehealth.com
- Iron, *easyIron*—Platinum: www.platinumnaturals.com
- Organika—full spectrum, plant enzymes for good digestion: www.organika.com
- *Bio-K+*, living probiotic cultures, preferred source, fermented yogurt medium, with 50 billion viable, active bacteria per 3.5 oz container: www.biokplus.com
- Probiotics, enteric-coated—Jarrow-EPS: www.jarrow.com, and Flora: www.florahealth.com
- Insulin regulation, *WellBetX*: www.naturalfactors.com and www.lef.org

- Maca powder (organic gelatinized)—Navitas naturals: www.navitasnaturals.com
- SAM-e 200 mg, timed release melatonin, stevia packets: www.naturesharmony.com
- Migraines, SISU *Petadolex®* butterbur extract: www.petadolex.ca
- Multi-vitamin-mineral formula, with nifty complete daily packs: www.questvitamins.com
- Melatonin, liquid, preferred source, *Natrol*: www.natrol.com
- Joint and muscle pain, *Atrosan gel*, fresh arnica gel: www.bioforce.ca
- GABA—Now: www.nowfoods.com
- Natural skin care products, *Dream Cream*, hand-made with care: www.aromacrystal.com
- L-theanine, 100 mg and R(+)-lipoic acid 100 mg: www.AOR.ca and www.lef.org
- B-12 sublingual 5 mg methylcobalamin: www.AOR.ca and www.lef.org.
- AllerSense, herbal extracts for ease of breathing, allergy relief: www.healthyimmunity.com
- Nutristart Vitamin Co., *Betty's Own*, 5 star rating, organic facial moisturizers and multi-purpose skin creams: (800) 813-4233 or www.nutristart.com

WELLNESS RESOURCES

The following alphabetical resource listings are both websites and telephone numbers for current health information, self-study courses, research results or to locate a health practitioner.

Alive Academy of Nutrition health advisor self-study: www.alive.com or (800) 663-6580

American Academy of Anti-Aging Medicine: www.worldhealth.net

American Association of Oriental Medicine: www.aaom.org

American Botanical Counsel—herbal newsletter: www.herbalgram.org

Berkeley Wellness newsletter: www.berkeleywellness.com

Calorie Restriction Society: www.calorierestriction.org

Canadian College of Naturopathic Medicine: www.ccnm.edu or (866) 241-2266

College Pharmacy—bio-identical hormones in the western U.S.: (800) 888-9358

Daybreak in My Soul—beautiful meditative songs for gamma synchrony: www.theforestofpeace.com

EEG—news, national list of EEG therapists and training programs: www.EEGspectrum.com

DORway—information on artificial sweeteners: www.dorway.com/blayenn.html

Esquimalt Peoples Pharmacy—Alan Hicke, MSc. Pharm, bio-identical hormone replacement compounding specialist in Canada: www.prescriptiondrugsonline.ca

Genuine Health—free *Health & Happiness* newsletter: www.genuinehealth.com

Grass-fed animals—list of farmers: www.eatwild.com and www.pasture-to-plate.com

Harvard Health letter: www.health.harvard.edu

Infrared saunas: www.infraredhealth.com or www.sunlightsaunas.com

Institute of HeartMath®: www.heartmath.com

International Academy of Compounding Pharmacists—natural hormone alternatives to hormone replacement therapy (HRT): (800) 927-4227

International Center for Metabolic Testing—complete blood and hormone testing in Canada: www.icmt.com or (888) 591-4124

Life Extension Magazine and Life Extension Update: www.lef.org or (800) 544-4440

Meditation CD "Toward Health and Wellness": www.towardstillness.com or (905) 820-4706

Nutrition and ORAC information on food: www.nal.usda.gov/fnic/foodcomp/search

Nutritional list of foods and fiber: www.fatfreekitchen.com/fiberlist

Magnetico—magnetic sleeping pads: www.magneticosleep.com

National Center for Complementary and Alternative Medicine—supplement information and "searchable" clinical trials: www.nccam.nih.gov

National Institutes of Health (NIH)—great free news on health at www.nih.gov

National Sleep Foundation—sleep information: www.sleepfoundation.org

Organic food information: www.consumersunion.org

Optimal breathing—articles and instructions: www.breathing.com

Tai Chi—books, videos, groups near you: www.taichifoundation.org and www.thetaichisite.com

The American Association of Naturopathic Physicians: www.naturopathic.org or (877) 969-2267

The Physicians and Sportsmedicine Online—great information on fitness and nutrition: www.physsportsmed.com

Townsend Letter for Doctors—alternative newsletter: www.townsend.com or (360) 385-6021

USDA Food Pyramid (1/m) revised in April 2005—www. mypyramid.gov

Women's Health Letter—by Nan K. Fuchs, PhD: www.womenshealthletter.com

Women's Health—National Women's Health Resource Center: www.healthywomen.org

World Health—HealthWorld Online, comprehensive information: www.healthy.net

REFERENCES

CHAPTER 1: FEELING GOOD IS GOOD FOR YOU

Cohen, G. *The Creative Age*. Avon Books Inc., New York, 2000.
Csikszentmihalyi, M. *Finding Flow*. Basic Books, New York, 1998.
Diener, E. Satisfaction with Life Scale. *Psychological Assessment*, Vol. 5, No. 2, 1993: 164–172.
Dossey, L. *Healing Words*. Harper Collins, San Francisco, 1993.
Hawkins, D.R. *Power vs. Force*. Hay House, Carlsbad, California, 2004.
Seligman, M. *Authentic Happiness*. Free Press, New York, 2002.
Warm, J. *Psychology of Perception*. Holt Kinehart, New York, 1999.
Williamson, M. *The Gift of Change*. Harper Collins, San Francisco, 2004.

CHAPTER 2: POSITIVE THINKING DOES MAKE YOU HAPPY

Beattie, M. *Codependent No More*. Hazeldon Educational Materials, Minnesota, 1992.
Cardoso, S.H. "Our Ancient Laughing Brain." *Cerebrum*. Dane Press, New York, Fall 2002.
Childre, D., and H. Martin. *The HeartMath Solution*. Harper Collins, San Francisco, 1999.
Myss, C. *Why People Don't Change*. Three Rivers Press, New York, 1997.
Restak, R. *The New Brain*. St. Martin's Press, New York, 2004.
Selye, H. *The Stress of Life*. McGraw-Hill, New York, 1978.

CHAPTER 3: ONE GREAT DAY *EQUALS* ONE GREAT LIFE

Benson, H. *The Relaxation Response*. Avon, New York, 1975.
Conrad, P. *Modern Times, Modern Places*. Alfred A. Knopf, New York, 1999.
Genazzani, A., Stomati M. "Long Term Low-Dose DHEA Oral Supplementation." *Fertility Sterility* 80 (6), Dec. 2003: 1495–1501.
Graci, S. *The Food Connection*. Macmillan, Toronto, 2001.
Helmuth, L. "Moral Reasoning Relies on Emotion." *Science*, 293, Sept. 14, 2001: 1971–1972.
Selye, H. *The Stress of Life*. McGraw-Hill, New York, 1978.

CHAPTER 4: WHAT SIGNALS ARE YOU SENDING TO YOUR BODY?

Barnard, N. *Breaking the Food Seduction.* St. Martin's Press, New York, 2003.

Brite, A. "What Are the Costs of Multitasking?" *Neurology Reviews,* 9.9, Sept. 2001: 59–60.

Graci, S. *The Food Connection.* Macmillan, Toronto, 2001.

Graci, S. *The Power of Superfoods.* Prentice Hall, Toronto, 1999.

King, B. *Fat Wars: 45 Days to Transform Your Body.* CDG Books Canada, Toronto, 2001.

Kurzweil, R., and T. Grossman. *Fantastic Voyage.* Rodale, Emmaus, Pennsylvania, 2004.

CHAPTER 5: TURN OFF YOUR ENERGY ZAPPERS

Andrus, C. *Simply...Woman!* Hay House, Carlsbad, California, 2004.

Applegate, L. *Eat Smart Play Hard.* Rodale, Emmaus, Pennsylvania, 2001.

Brink, Susan. "Sleepless Society." *U.S. News and World Report,* Oct. 16, 2000.

Schmidt, M.A. *Smart Fats.* Frog Ltd., Berkeley, California, 1997.

Shulman, J. *Winning the Food Fight.* John Wiley & Sons, Toronto, 2003.

CHAPTER 6: DOWNSHIFT YOUR TASTE BUDS AND YOUR LIFE

Dyer, W. *10 Secrets for Success and Inner Peace.* Hay House, Carlsbad, California, 2001.

Hendricks, G. *Achieving Vibrance.* Harmony Books, New York, 2002.

Stedman, G. *You Can Make It Happen: A 9-Step Plan for Success.* Fireside Books, New York, 1997.

CHAPTER 7: FOOD AS MEDICINE—CELL-FRIENDLY EATING

Boon, H. et al. "The Effects of greens+." *Journal of Dietetic Practice and Research,* August 2004.

Rao, V. "The Invitro and Invivo Antioxidant Effects of greens+." *Journal of Medicinal Foods,* Fall 2005.

CHAPTER 8: TEST-DRIVE THE SEVEN-DAY REJUVENATION PLAN

Alarcon de la Lastra, et al. "Mediterranean Diet and Health: Olive Oil." *Current Pharmaceutical*, July 2001.

Cutler, R.G. "Antioxidants and Aging." *American Journal of Clinical Nutrition*, Vol. 53, 1999: 373–379.

Heshka, J., and P. Jones. "A Role for Dietary Fat in Leptin Receptors." *Life Science*, 2001: 987–1003.

Simopoulos, A.P., V. Herbert, and B. Jacobson. *Genetic Nutrition: Designing a Diet Based on Your Family Medical History*. Macmillan Publishing Co., New York, 1993.

Vanderhaeghe, L.R., and K. Karst. *Healthy Fats for Life*. Quarry Health Books, Kingston, 2003.

CHAPTER 9: FOUR TIPS TO ENERGIZE YOUR DAY—TODAY!

Burns, D.D. *Feeling Good*. Avon Books Inc., New York, 1999.

Kalmijn, S. et al. "Dietary Intake of Fatty Acids and Fish in Relation to Cognitive Performance at Middle Age." *Neurology*, Jan. 2004: 275–280.

Stevens, L. et al. "Fish Oils ADD/ADHD." *Lipids*, 2003.

CHAPTER 11: EAT IN TUNE WITH YOUR GENETIC CODE

Cutler, R.G. "Antioxidants and Aging." *American Journal of Clinical Nutrition*, Vol. 53, 1999: 373–379.

Schneider, L., and F. Garland. "Sunlight, Vitamin D, and Ovarian Cancer." *International Journal of Epidemiology*, Vol. 23, No. 6, Dec. 1994: 1133–1136.

Suzuki, M., B. Wilcox, and C. Wilcox. "Implications from and for Food Cultures for Cardiovascular Disease: Longevity." *Asia Pacific Journal of Clinical Research*, 10(2), 2001: 165–171.

Terman, A. "Garbage Catastrophe Theory of Aging: Imperfect Removal of Oxidative Damage?" *Redox*, 2001: 6C, 15–26.

Wickelgren, I. "Tracking Insulin to the Mind." *Science*, 280, 1998: 517–522.

CHAPTER 12: BEYOND CLEANSING: DAILY DETOX

Bland, J., and S. Benum. *The 20-Day Rejuvenation Diet Program.* Keats Publishing Inc. New Canaan, Connecticut, 1999.

Brown, A., ed. *Present Knowledge in Nutrition.* 6th ed. : International Life Science Foundation, Washington, D.C.,1990.

Northrup, C. *The Wisdom of Menopause.* Bantam Books, New York, 2003.

Yeager, S. et al., eds. Prevention's *New Foods for Healing.* Rodale Press, Emmaus, Pennsylvania, 1998.

CHAPTER 13: SPIRITUAL INSIGHTS: BE INSPIRED

Ladinsky, D. *I Heard God Laughing—Renderings of Hafix.* Sufism Reoriented, Walnut Creek, California, 1996.

Langer, E. *Mindfulness.* Perseus Books, Reading, Mass., 1989.

Provine, R. *Laughter: A Scientific Investigation.* Penguin Books, New York, 2000.

Tiburon, A. *Course in Miracles.* Foundation for Inner Peace, Los Angeles, 1995.

Vardey, L. *The Flowering of the Soul, A Book of Prayers by Women.* Alfred A. Knopf, Toronto, 1999.

CHAPTER 14: TWENTY-ONE WAYS TO TWEAK YOUR LIFESTYLE

Baker, D. *What Happy People Know: How the New Science of Happiness Can Change Your Life for the Better.* St. Martin's Griffin, New York, 2004.

Cherniske, S. *The Metabolic Plan.* Ballantine Books, 2003.

Hanley, Jesse Lynn. *Tired of Being Tired.* Penguin Putnam, 2000.

Levine, P. *Walking the Tiger.* North Atlantic Books, 1997.

Natural Medicines Comprehensive Database: www.naturaldatabase.com

CHAPTER 15: TWENTY-ONE DAYS FROM ORDINARY TO REMARKABLE

Enig, M.G. *Know Your Fats.* Bethesda Press, Silver Springs, Maryland, 2000.

Graci, S. *The Food Connection.* Macmillan, Toronto, 2001.

Graci, S. *The Power of Superfoods.* Prentice Hall, Toronto, 1999.

Hyman, M., and M. Liponis. *Ultra Prevention*. Scribner, New York, 2003.
Weff, C. *Conscious Cuisine*. Sourcebooks, Inc., Naperville, Illinois, 2002.
Wurtman, R.J., and J.J. Wurtman. "Brain Serotonin Carbohydrate Craving, Obesity and Depression." *Obesity*, Nov. 1995, Suppl. 4: 477–480.

CHAPTER 16: IN PURSUIT OF HUMAN EXCELLENCE—MIGHTY BRAIN MESSENGERS

Braverman, E. *The Edge Effect*, Sterling Publishing, New York, 2004.
McCrone, J. "Right Brain or Left Brain: Myth or Reality?" *The New Scientist*, 2000.
Restak, R. *The Secret Life of the Brain*. The Dana Press and Joseph Heury Press, New York, 2001.
Rosenzweig, E.S. et al. "Making Room for New Memories." *Nature Neuroscience*, 5(1) 2002: 6–8.
Small, G. *The Memory Bible*. Hypericon, New York, 2002.
Small, G. *The Memory Prescription*. Hypericon, New York, 2004.
Taylor, S.E. *The Tending Instinct*. Henry Holt and Co., New York, 2001.

CHAPTER 17: IN PURSUIT OF HUMAN EXCELLENCE—THE MIND-BODY CONNECTION

Fotuhi, M. *The Memory Cure*. McGraw Hill, New York, 2003.
Johnson, S. *Mind Wide Open*. Scribner, New York, 2004.
Restak, R. *The New Brain*. Rodale, Emmaus, Pennsylvania, 2003.
Sellmeyer, D.E. et al. "A High Ratio of Dietary Animal to Vegetable Protein." *American Journal of Clinical Nutrition*, 73(1) Jan. 2001: 118–122.
Terry, R.D., and R. Katzman. "Lifespan and Synapses." *Neurobiology of Aging*, 22(3) 2001: 347–348.
Wisneski, L.A., and L. Anderson. *The Scientific Basis of Integrative Medicine*. CRC Press, New York, 2005.
Wright, R. *Non Zero: The Logic of Human Destiny*. Pantheon Books, New York, 2000.

CHAPTER 18: IN PURSUIT OF HUMAN EXCELLENCE—BE HEALTHY...BE HAPPY!

Ames, B.N. et al. "Are Vitamin and Mineral Deficiencies a Major Cancer Risk?" *Nat. Rev. Cancer*, Sept. 2002.

Ball, P. "Chemists Build Body Fluid Battery." *Nature Science*, Nov. 2002.

Lammers, D. "Micro Medical Devices Could Transform Health Care." *EE Times*, June 21, 2002.

Lombard, J., and C. Germano. *The Brain Wellness Plan*. Kensington Pub. Corp., New York, 2000.

Shultz, B. "The Developing Brain." *Scientific American*, 1992, Sept. 267: 60-67.

Vince, G. "Nanotechnology May Create New Organs." *New Scientist*, July 8, 2003.

Whitfield, J. "Lasers Operate Inside Single Cells." *Nature Science Update*, Oct. 6, 2003.

Wilson, R.S. et al. "Depressive Symptoms, Cognitive Decline and Risk of AD in Older Persons." *Neurology*, 59(3), 2002: 364–370.

INDEX